THE GREATEST
EXPERIMENT
EVER PERFORMED
ON WOMEN

THE GREATEST EXPERIMENT EVER PERFORMED ON WOMEN

Exploding the Estrogen Myth

BARBARA SEAMAN

HYPERION

New York

"The Coming of Wisdom With Time" by W.B. Yeats, from *The Collected Works of W.B. Yeats, Volume I: The Poems, Revised*, edited by Richard J. Finneran (New York: Scribner, 1997).

ISBN 0-7868-6853-8

Hyperion books are available for special promotions and premiums. For details contact Michael Rentas, Manager, Inventory and Premium Sales, Hyperion, 77 West 66th Street, 11th floor, New York, New York 10023, or call 212-456-0133.

FIRST EDITION

10 9 8 7 6 5 4 3 2 1

This book is in appreciation of my children
Noah, Elana, Shira

And my grandchildren
Sophia, Idalia, Liam, and Ezekiel

There's No Free Lunch, But There's Free Dessert

ACKNOWLEDGMENTS

PUBLISHING: To Valerie Borchardt, my calm and delightful agent, and to Leigh Haber, my Hyperion editor, a canary-in-the-mine at sensing upcoming topics, a tiger at getting them into print.

To Ben Loehnen, Leigh Haber's crackerjack assistant, and Cassie M. Meyer, who preceded him.

To Christine Ragasa, a careful and trustworthy publicist.

HOMEFRONT: To Laura Eldridge, my intern from Barnard College, writer, editor, critic, original thinker, who helped me begin this book and who stayed on after graduation to see it through.

To Agata Rumprecht at SUNY Stony Brook, who sharpened my pencils and practiced her English here as a little girl from Poland, and who grew up into an accomplished researcher and witty writer.

Additional thanks to Maria Tylutka, Lauren Gmitter, Tatiana Rios, Tim Partridge, Elka Krajewska, Edward Stern, and Timothy Walsh, Esq.

NATIONAL INSTITUTES OF HEALTH: To Vivian Pinn, M.D., Office of Research on Women's Health, and Jacques Rossouw, M.D.,

Women's Health Initiative; to Sylvia Smoller, Ph.D., and all the Principal Investigators, and their staffs, and to the volunteers who laid their bodies on the line. To Loretta Finnegan, M.D., and Ellen Pollack in Dr. Pinn's office. To a new era, where treatment choices are based on evidence, and where patients, and doctors, learn to tell a reliable study from smoke and mirrors.

OTHERS AT THE NIH: To C.W. (Bill) Jameson, Ph.D., National Institute of Environmental Health Science; James Lacey, Ph.D., National Cancer Institute; Sherry Sherman, Ph.D., National Institute on Aging.

FDA: To Philip Corfman, M.D. (retired), Suzanne Parisian, M.D. (author of FDA: Inside and Out), Bruce Stadel, M.D., Susan Wood, Ph.D., Lisa Rarick, M.D.

FDA HISTORY OFFICE: Suzanne White Junod, Ph.D., John Swann, Ph.D.

LIBRARY OF CONGRESS: Frederick W. Bauman.

CONGRESS: Hon. Carolyn Maloney of New York, and Minna Elias and Robin Bachman.

U.S. DEPARTMENT OF HEALTH AND HUMAN SERVICES: Donna Shalala, Ph.D., Sarah Kovner.

ACADEMIA AND OTHER EXPERT CONSULTANTS AND SOURCES: Jean Jofen, Ph.D. (psychology); Diana Petitti, M.D. (epidemiology); Pat Cody of DES–Action (archivist of early estrogen and cancer studies, and of past and present information on effects of diethylstilbestrol); Elizabeth Siegel Watkins, Ph.D. (history); Carl Djerassi, Ph.D. (history); Robert Proctor, Ph.D. (history); David Endo (alternative medicine); Adrienne Fugh-Berman, M.D. (alternative medicine); Pat Crawshaw (osteoporosis); Carol Ann Rinzler (breast cancer); Alison Abbott (history); Lila Wallis, M.D. (osteoporosis); Harry K. Genant, M.D. (osteoporosis); John C. LaRosa, M.D. (heart); Naomi Rogers, Ph.D. (history);

Charles Debrovner, M.D. (tapering off estrogen); Harriet Presser, Ph.D. (demography); Larry Sasich (pharmacy and pharmacology); Molly Ginty (sea of estrogens); Barron Lerner, M.D. (cancer politics); Ulf Schmidt (history); Donald T. Critchlow (history); Lara Marks, Ph.D. (history); and Sidney Wolfe, M.D.

WOMEN'S HEALTH RIGHTS: Cynthia Pearson; Judy Norsigian; Amy Allina; Susan Love, M.D.; Mary Ann Napoli; Sheryl Burt Ruzek, Ph.D.; Anne Rochon Ford; Sharon Batt; Belita Cowan; Shere Hite; Phyllis Chesler, Ph.D.; Paula Caplan, Ph.D.; Ann Kasper, Ph.D.; Byllye Avery; Alice Wolfson, Esq.; Oliva Cousins, Ph.D.

EXPERT READERS AND MANUSCRIPT REVIEW: Myra Appleton; Urs Bamert (German translations); Jennifer Baumgardner (history); Jessica Baumgardner; Devra Lee Davis, Ph.D. (sea of estrogens); Michael Patrick Hearn (history); Fredi Kronenberg, Ph.D. (alternative treatments); Kathryn Scarbrough, Ph.D. (Alzheimer's); Noah Seaman; Ann O'Shea (sea of estrogens); Andrea Tone, Ph.D. (history); Betsy Wade.

CORPORATE HISTORIES: Joe Ciccone, Corporate Archivist, Merck & Co; Kim Schillace, Berlex Labs; Christine Berghausen, Andre Schmolke, Wolfgang Frobenious, Schering; Stephen Simes, Biosante and Searle; Lois A. Gaeta, Ayerst Laboratories.

AMERICAN MEDICAL ASSOCIATION: Drummond Rennie, M.D.; Roy Schwarz, M.D. (retired); Harriet Meyer, M.D.; Ron Davis, M.D.

INDEPENDENT MEDICAL SOURCES: No Free Lunch listserve, Biojest Listserve, National Women's Health Network, Health Research Group.

DR. ROBERT GREENBLATT: Edward Greenblatt, Esq.; Deborah Greenblatt; Virendra B. Mahesh, Ph.D.; Paul McDonough, M.D.

DR. ROBERT WILSON: Ronald Wilson.

MADELINE GRAY: Roger Kahn, Sylvia Seaman.

PROVIDERS OF INFORMATION, DOCUMENTS, INTRO-DUCTIONS, AND OTHER SUPPORT: Nikki Scheuer; Sheila Bandman and Donald Bandman: Judith Rossner and Stanley Leff; Myrna and Jeffrey Blyth; Audrey Flack and Bob Marcus; Maria and Norman Marcus; Judge Emily Jane Goodman; Daniel Simon; Shere Hite; Alix Kates Shulman; Letty Cottin Pogrebin; Jacqui Ceballos; Marlene Sanders; Mary Jean Tully; William Klein; Deborah Chase; Lucy Komisar; Grace Petti; Ernest, Jeri, and Jense Drucker; Elaine, Pablo, and Henry Rosner–Jeria; Ruth Gruber; and Joanna Perlman for her Over the Rainbow work on the Appendix.

HADASSAH MAGAZINE: Joan Michel, Alan Tigay, Zelda Shluker, and the readers who write in.

MS. MAGAZINE: Gloria Steinem

NEW YORK TIMES AND WASHINGTON POST: Alex Ward

PROJECT CENSORED: Peter Phillips

EXTRA: Jim Naureckas

IN MEMORIAM:

TWO SAINTS

Mary Howell, M.D. (d. 1998), and Helen Rodriguez-Trias, M.D. (d. 2001), my dear colleagues who worked tirelessly for the rights of patients, of minorities, of women in medicine, and, being pediatricians, for all children everywhere. Howell was a cofounder of the National Women's Health Network. Rodriguez-Trias was a longtime president of the Board: *"The women's movement is about survival, about finding our strength and using it to help other women. We reach out to each other to build a different kind of society—one where women are equal in power to men and where children are truly prized."*

—Dr. Helen Rodriguez-Trias in *The Conversation Begins*, by Christina Loper Baker and Christina Baker Kline.

THREE WISE MENTORS

Peter Wyden (d. 1998), my editor at the *Ladies' Home Journal* and, later, publisher of *The Doctors' Case against the Pill* (1969). An immigrant from Germany, when he returned with the U.S. Army after World War II as a specialist in "information control" he investigated reports that hormonal contraceptives were tested in Auschwitz.

Victor Cohn (d. 2000), author of *News and Numbers*, was Science Editor of the *Minneapolis Tribune* and then the *Washington Post*. In his generation, he was the most respected journalist in his field, the "Dean." Author of a column called "The Patients' Advocate," when *The Doctors' Case against the Pill* was published he exposed the campaign by manufacturers and population control organizations to discredit it.

Sir Edward Charles Dodds (d. 1973) discovered the first popular low-cost estrogen that was effective by mouth, diethylstilbestrol, but worried that it was used too casually and for too long. In 1945, he reported that "disturbing symptoms of menopause" could be successfully treated as follows: "It is found that if estrogens are administered to the patient in decreasing amounts over a period of about one year, the symptoms are suppressed during the course of the therapy and do not recur when it is fully discontinued." He did add, "There are individual variations in the time," but his message was that *one year of therapy was ample for most women and that in starting a very slow taper as soon as the symptoms were under control, recurrence at the other end could be prevented.*

CONTENTS

CONTENTS

Contents

THE GREATEST
EXPERIMENT
EVER PERFORMED
ON WOMEN

PART I

HOW DID ALL THIS HAPPEN?

Introduction I: Smart Doctors, Foolish Forecasts

I have a doctor friend who so believed in the value of synthetic estrogens that when the National Institutes of Health announced a large clinical trial to compare these pills with sugar pills, she dismissed it as a waste of money. "Obviously, the women on the hormones will be living longer," she said. "It's unethical to leave volunteers on the placebos for the full eight and a half years of the trial. At some point they'll have to stop the study and offer hormones to everyone."

Her colleagues concurred, but then the opposite came true. On the morning of July 9, 2002, my friend, along with other physicians and the 30 million U.S. patients taking estrogen products, woke up to discover that the world, after all, was flat. A safety-monitoring board had suddenly halted a part of the study involving 16,608 women because those taking hormones had more breast cancer, heart attacks, strokes, pulmonary embolisms, and blood clots than those taking sugar pills. Yes, the volunteers on Prempro also had fewer bone fractures and less colon cancer. But not enough to balance out the risks.

My friend initially heard the startling results on *Good Morning America*, where Dr. Tim Johnson described this "somewhat surprising outcome." He predicted that most women then taking hormone pills would stop "after talking to their physicians today," failing to anticipate that many doctors would take their telephones off the hook. My friend switched the channel to CNN, where Paula Zahn repeatedly exclaimed: "I tell you— women gotta go insane today." Channel surfing, my friend caught up with the "usual suspects," certain doctors familiar to TV viewers whose spin skills had been developed by public-relations coaches at agencies that handle pharmaceutical accounts. It was then that my friend got it. These physicians were appearing on stations where paid ads suggested that if only we took estrogen we could look like Lauren Hutton and sing like Patti LaBelle.

That night my friend called me to apologize for having objected to the title I planned for this book. She had called it "over the top and ridiculous," but now she said she could almost agree.

WHAT IS THE GREATEST EXPERIMENT?

While the Prempro arm of the Women's Health Initiative, which lasted 5.2 years and included 16,608 women, was a major test, it is only a small part of what I consider to be *The Greatest Experiment Ever Performed on Women*. The experiment began in England in 1938, and it has continued for sixty-five years. A British biochemist, desperate to prevent Nazi Germany from cornering the world market on synthetic sex hormones, published his formula for cheap and powerful oral estrogen. Within months, thousands of doctors and scores of drug companies around the world were working with this formula.

That opened the Greatest Experiment. Products made from chemicals that mimicked the feminizing effects of a woman's natural secretions were marketed fresh out of the lab. They were prescribed and sold for a host of concerns—to slow and prevent aging, to stop hot flashes, to avoid pregnancy or miscarriage, and as a morning-after contraceptive.

I call the marketing, prescribing, and sale of these drugs an experiment because, for all these years, they have been used, in the main, for what doctors and scientists hope or believe they can do, not for what they *know* the products can do. Medical policy on estrogens has been to "shoot first and apologize later"—to prescribe the drugs for a certain health problem and then see if there is a positive result. Over the years, hundreds of millions, possibly billions of women, have been lab animals in this unofficial trial. They were not volunteers. They were given no consent forms. And they were put at serious, often devastating risk.

The risks of these drugs have been known and documented from the start. The British doctor who published his estrogen formula in 1938 spent many years thereafter warning the world that these drugs, although containing great promise, put women at serious peril for endometrial and breast cancer. Since the halting of the Prempro trial in July, despite the ignorance or hypocrisy of many doctors who said "Who knew?," there is nothing surprising in the recent findings. We have known since day one that these drugs posed threats. And since then science has added to, not subtracted from, the list of estrogen's problems.

If doctors and scientists have known these dirty secrets for so long, why is the bad press so recent? That is an essential question right now, and this book seeks to present the answer. Part of the answer lies in the vigorous efforts by drug companies to protect an invaluable market. These efforts have included underwriting studies and subsidizing doctors, participating in medical-school curriculums, advertising heavily in medical journals, and seeing that continuing medical education is directed by doctors on the drug industry's payroll. They have also entailed one of the most elaborate promotion and advertising campaigns in the history of the media not only in America but worldwide.

This is not the first time estrogen sales have felt the cold wind of consumer anger. In 1975, the magnitude of estrogen-related endometrial cancer was established; drug sales sank by half in subsequent years. In that instance, as in every other that has cast suspicion on estrogen, the drug companies managed to revitalize sales through new claims, which is why I say that only through learning how these companies buy and influence medical opinion can women protect themselves from any new spin, any new claim that will inevitably emerge about these drugs and countless others.

Estrogen products won't go away, and they shouldn't. One can only wish, as I do, that they will be used now with caution, based on evidence and facts, not illusion. My aim is to consider whether hormone supplements are necessary and for whom. Specifically, I hope this book will help women navigate the estrogen issue and keep anything similar from happening again. But the larger hope is that we can make informed decisions about other drugs as well.

On the sixty-fifth birthday of the Greatest Experiment, I recall a poem by William Butler Yeats entitled "The Coming of Wisdom with Time":

> *Though leaves are many, the root is one;*
> *Through all the lying days of my youth*
> *I swayed my leaves and flowers in the sun*
> *Now I may wither into the truth.*

Let us hope.

CHAPTER 1

ON THE PATH TO PREMARIN

If a menopausal woman has pain or makes trouble, pound her hard
on the jaw.

— EGYPTIAN MEDICAL TEXT, 2000 B.C.

More than five hundred years ago, a medical book from Renais-
sance Europe recommended that the woman having problems in
menopause receive "a decoction of myrrh and apples." If that didn't work,
"a cure may sometimes also be affected by pouring some of this same substance into her sandals, and urging the patient to walk." In effect, the remedy was an herbal one—mixed with exercise.

Nowadays the American Medical Association (AMA) reports that half
of the adults in the United States are using or have used health treatments
derived from plants, called herbals or botanicals, for all manner of conditions. Many of these substances are pharmacologically active, and
some—such as echinacea—have remained popular for hundreds, even

thousands, of years. What are less well known and often left unspoken (being repugnant to some people) are medicines derived from animals, particularly their organs and their secretions, yet animal parts have been used in health care through the ages, some of them for the purpose of easing menopause complaints. One such medicine, featured in the *Merck Manual* for 1899, was a coarse brownish powder called Ovariin, available in pills flavored with vanillin or in tablet form. Ovariin was prescribed for "climacterica," also known as menopause, and other "ills" referable to the ovaries. Gruesomely enough, Ovariin was derived from the dried and pulverized ovaries of a cow. The recommended dose was 8 to 24 grains three times daily.

I queried Dr. Jacques Rossouw, director of the NIH Women's Health Initiative, on whether he supposed that the cow-ovary product could have been biologically active. "Yes," he replied, "I do think that the dried cow's ovary would have been somewhat effective taken orally. Steroid hormones are pretty robust and would survive drying and powdering, but I suspect that only a small portion would be absorbed from the intestines. Injection would be needed for high efficacy." Dr. Rossouw's conclusion: Ovariin may have had some estrogenic effect.

It's nice to know that this early product wasn't snake oil, but the most striking thing about Ovariin is that Merck was already selling animal-based estrogen treatments more than a century ago. After all, it is part of the canon of doctors and writers who push hormones that menopause is a phenomenon of the modern age. Until now, they proclaim positively, few women survived long enough to "outlive their ovaries." But if menopause is a function of today's longevity and good diet, why would a nineteenth-century *Merck Manual* recommend Ovariin, not to mention a choice of twenty-eight additional treatments for woman's climacteric?

The answer lies in coming to grips with a modern misinterpretation of old medical statistics. In the nineteenth century, the average life expectancy of a newborn baby girl was the early to mid-forties — if, that is, she wasn't the one in five who would not survive past her first birthday. The mother faced a one in forty chance of dying in the process of giving birth. But even then, the fact was that if a baby girl born in the nineteenth century got safely to the end of her childbearing years, she could claim a remaining life span almost equal to what we have today. So why do we accept that before the twentieth century, few women made it to menopause? Because when we look at statistics from the nineteenth century (or earlier) showing a lower age of death, we forget we are looking at an average that includes many individuals who died very young, balancing out those who lived threescore and ten years or longer.

Given the former perils of the female reproductive years, it's not surprising that some women and their doctors viewed menstruation as an illness and a burden, while welcoming menopause as a triumph. Menopause is not a new phenomenon, nor is seeing it as a period of adjustment rather than a disease. A century and a half ago, the "change" was written about in validating terms. "After a certain number of years, woman lays aside those functions with which she has been endowed for the perpetuation of the species, and resumes once more that exclusively individual life which has been hers when a child," wrote George Napheys in his charming 1869 book *The Physical Life of Woman: Advice to the Maiden, Wife, and Mother.* "The evening of her days approaches, and if she has observed the precepts of wisdom, she may look forward to a long and placid period of rest, blessed with health, honored and loved with a purer flame than any which she inspired in the bloom of youth and beauty."

Napheys hailed from Canada, but across the Atlantic were like-minded French society physicians who referred to menopause positively as *le retour d'age*, meaning a return to youth before the times of fertility, a return to more carefree days. In the spirit of viewing menopause as the opportunity for a woman to vigorously reclaim her own life, many doctors urged their patients to avoid harsh medicines, as hot flashes "were natural and not an illness." In *The Diseases of Females* (1837), Thomas Graham sounds quite contemporary when he presses the point that except for attention to diet and exercise, "little or nothing is required for the management of ordinary cases."

GETTING HIGH ON MENOPAUSE

The modern story of menopause treatment can be traced to Merck, a high-class, high-volume purveyor of pharmaceuticals. The Merck family had been proprietors since 1668 of a stylish apothecary in Darmstadt, Germany. Though always successful, they did not secure their great fortune until the nineteenth century, when in 1827, Heinrich Emanuel Merck achieved "the first manufacture" on a commercial scale of morphine. Codeine followed in 1836, and cocaine in 1862—handily "taking the business from pharmacy to factory." Thus, along with powdered ovaries from cows, the 1899 *Merck Manual* could offer the woman who was "undone" or "unstrung" by menopause a panoply of products to ease her days and nights. She might choose among amyl nitrate, belladonna, cannabis, and the best-selling Merck Opium U.S.P., this last offered in a fine selection of delivery systems and bases, including wine, vinegar, liquorice troches, and orange peel, either bitter or sweet. In 1897 the price for fifty tablets of Ovariin was $1.25; the pharmacist would pay $8.00 for just one ounce. Opium was considerably cheaper, the pharmacist being charged only $4.00 per pound.

Besides providing the narcotics to "ease" menopausal symptoms,

Merck was an innovator in capitalizing on the use of animal glands in medicine. History records that the sex glands of animals were employed (often controversially) as an aphrodisiac, youth tonic, and fertility booster, and to ease the symptoms of menopause by health providers (sometimes regarded as witches or devils) in various cultures over many thousands of years. We also know exactly when such treatments took a sharp turn toward respectability and gained consideration as "serious science." It was June in Paris, 1889, when Charles Edouard Brown-Sequard, a beloved and admired seventy-two-year-old doctor, reported he had "rejuvenated himself" by injecting extracts from guinea pig and dog testicles into "sensitive parts of his body." Dr. Brown-Sequard's claims prompted many scientists to explore the properties of other reproductive organs and their secretions.

Brown-Sequard's lecture regarding his exploits was translated into English by a very interested twentieth-century science writer by the name of Madeline Gray (more on Madeline Gray later). "Messieurs," Dr. Brown-Sequard said, "all my life, as you know, I have been a hard worker. But lately my strength, which was at one time great, has considerably diminished. Up until two weeks ago I was so weak I had to sit down instead of stand in the laboratory. And when I got home, all I could do was partake of a meager supper and go straight to bed." He went on to explain that to counteract this unfamiliar lethargy he had begun giving himself a series of injections. He had removed the sex glands from some young and energetic dogs, boiled the glands down into a concentrate, and injected this concentrate into himself. "Behold the results!" he continued. "After only a few injections I can work for hours. I stand up in the laboratory instead of sitting down. And when I get home, I eat a hearty supper and return once more to my work." As he tinkered with and further perfected his mixture of guinea pig and dog testicle extracts, Brown-Sequard began to sound like a preview of some of today's more extreme advocates of hormone replace-

had pitched in to follow up the work of Allen and Doisy, sometimes vaulting the new hurdles a step or two ahead of their predecessors.

Hormone research was hot, a frontier not just for science but for its Jekyll-and-Hyde counterpart, the development of new drugs for market. Easing the financial way for some researchers, drug manufacturers dreamed about new hormone product lines. They thought menopause. They thought menstruation. They thought beautiful skin, thicker hair, more passionate sex. They thought of curing infertility, preventing miscarriages, and drying up breast milk in mothers who preferred to bottle-feed. Some of the more daring were also thinking birth control. Records indicate that at least two companies, Schering in Germany and Richter in Hungary, had figured out formulas for oral contraceptives before the start of World War II, although it wouldn't be until 1960 that the pill was made generally available.

With visions of future profits dancing in their heads, drug manufacturers went out scouting, like college recruiters seeking high school talent for their sports teams. With open checkbooks, they courted young biochemists in particular. Some of the very greatest young scientists accepted their patronage, including Canada's James Bertram Collip, who'd produced the first insulin suitable for use in human beings in January 1922. The father of insulin went on to become the father of Premarin as well. In Germany, Adolph Butenandt, who was unable to pick up his Nobel Prize in 1939 because Hitler personally forbade him to leave the country, was provided his raw materials (such as human urine) by the Schering company. Even the late-pregnancy urine of German women used for his estrogen research and the urine of officers from the Berlin police barracks used for his work on testosterone were procured by the giant German pharmaceutical firm. Not everyone chased the drug industry carrot, though. The English genius Edward Charles Dodds was scouted by Eli Lilly and other U.S. firms, but in the end he declined their offers and carried on his definitive estrogen research on behalf of his own laboratory, Courtauld Institute of Biochemistry, at London's Middlesex Hospital.

Edgar Allen, the man who opened the door to female hormones, continued his research in the field. In 1933, Allen accepted an invitation to chair the anatomy department at Yale Medical School. Allen and Doisy kept up some of their work together. Allen was getting more into research on the role of estrogens in female cancers, while Doisy was focusing on vitamins, and in 1939 they coauthored a definitive book, descriptively titled *Sex and Internal Secretions*. In April 1941, just as the FDA was examining applications from Eli Lilly, Squibb, and several other companies to approve estrogen products for the treatment of menopause, Allen published an article in the journal *Cancer Research* on the propensity of estrogens to cause cervical cancer in animals. *"Estrogen is a very important factor, not merely an incidental one, in cervical carcinogenesis,"* Allen and his coauthor concluded. This statement was a breakthrough—estrogen is a carcinogen!—but it fell on deaf ears. Hormones were such a promising pharmaceutical, nobody wanted to hear that those years of industry-funded research might have yielded a drug women should not take.

Nobody, that is, except for the cancer experts Michael Shimkin, a founder of the National Cancer Institute; Charles Dodds, who had discovered the very estrogen the drug companies were trying to get approved; and George Papanicolaou, inventor of the Pap smear, a method for the early detection of cervical cancer. The real cancer experts all listened to Allen's warning, but what did that matter when so much money was at stake?

By 1942, one year after Allen's declaration that estrogen could cause cancer, Premarin, an estrogen made from the urine of pregnant mares, was put on the market by Ayerst Laboratories. It was an instant hit and has remained one of the most enduring and profitable drugs in history.

The first time I ever heard the word *Premarin* was at the deathbed of my aunt Sally, who had endometrial cancer. It was 1959. Sally was my father's twin and my official second mother, since Sally had no children of her own. She was just short of her fiftieth birthday when we gathered around her oxygen tent on a ward at Memorial Hospital, New York City's famous center for cancer treatment.

Sally's sisters and nieces were in attendance. A devoted young doctor who had been on her case from the beginning came by to check on her frequently. After he got to know us, he pulled the female relatives aside and indicated that he wished to tell us something. It was about estrogen. "Don't take it. Please don't ever take it," he said. "You are Sally's sisters and nieces. You may have the same susceptibilities."

I was dumbstruck by how passionate he was on this topic. I was fresh out of Oberlin College and had just begun writing about women's health, so I was curious and skeptical, too. I asked the doctor how he could be so certain that Sally's cancer came from Premarin.

From the appearance of the lawless pattern of cells in the lining of her uterus, her endometrium, he said. That estrogen was to endometrial cancer what cigarettes are to lung cancer had been reported by Dr. Saul Gusberg in 1947, but I didn't know that yet, nor did the vast majority of women taking estrogen. "It's a special cancer. An estrogen cancer. Your aunt told me that she doesn't blame her GP," the young doctor said. "She had severe hot flashes and night sweats. She begged him for the Premarin. But," he continued, "I fault him for letting her stay on it too long. The worst hot flashes in the world couldn't compare with what is happening to her now."

I gazed at my aunt, once adorably plump and round-faced, now shrunken to less than sixty pounds, suffused with pain—and I agreed. I heeded the warning of Sally's doctor. I never did take estrogen in any form, which makes me a little bit unusual. Any time I have been tempted (by the convenience of the birth control pill or Premarin's claims to be a fountain of youth), I remember that sweet young doctor who had feared for Aunt Sally's relatives.

I was twenty-three when Sally died, just starting out as a freelance magazine writer on women's health and sexuality. When we came back from the cemetery, I opened a file entitled "Premarin and Cancer." I still have the file. All these years I have watched and reported on the growing popularity of female hormone products. And all these years I have watched the rate of female cancers rise in lockstep with the sales.

CHAPTER 2

FOUNTAIN OF YOUTH OR
GOLDEN FLEECE?

Unlike my aunt Sally, who died of her menopause treatment, nobody I know of ever died of menopause, despite the fact that millions of miserable women may have wished they could. In her 1951 best-seller, *The Changing Years*, Madeline Gray lamented that "nature throws the book at the menopausal woman." Envying friends who had "no trouble at all," Madeline herself was "physically swept away as by lightning."

It was a great day when Madeline discovered Premarin. "I learned that prolonged menopausal suffering is almost unnecessary, since there is now, for the first time in history, 'blessed menopausal medicine' to help. Our mothers may have had to suffer—not us." Premarin was developed in Canada in the 1930s, and was approved by the FDA for treatment of menopause symptoms in 1942. Following her hysterectomy, Madeline remained on the "blessed" medicine for three years, sometimes sucking on testosterone lozenges for enhancement.

Due in part to *The Changing Years*, Gray's book, Premarin went on to become the twentieth century's biggest-selling brand-name prescription drug.

How Premarin Happened

In 1922, as a visitor in a Toronto laboratory run by Drs. Frederick Banting, C. H. Best, and J. J. R. Macleod, biochemist James Bertram "Bert" Collip produced the first insulin suitable for use in human beings. The creation of insulin was a great triumph of modern endocrinology, and one of the most lifesaving miracles in all of medical history. Although Collip was the newest and at age twenty-nine the most junior member of the research team, he was also the most instrumental. Yet within the year, after numerous bitter arguments, Collip left the project, returning to his teaching duties in Alberta. But his name (along with Drs. Banting and Best) remained on the insulin patent. In 1923, when Banting and Macleod received the Nobel Prize, Macleod gave the most deserving Collip a quarter share of the money. The *Canadian Encyclopedia* describes Collip, who died in 1965, as "the best scientist on the insulin team," and notes that afterwards he "made the most significant contributions to medical research. He did not court honors and seldom discussed the discovery of insulin."

As of this writing, some eighty years have passed, but Canadians still talk about how the Nobel Prize was stolen from young Collip. His further achievements in hormone research are extensive. He soon isolated the parathyroid hormone and in 1928 was appointed professor of biochemistry at McGill in Montreal. Then, for the following decade, he and his students "pioneered the isolation and study of the ovarian and gonadotrophic hormones"—until, when duty called, he packed it all in for wartime medical research.

Shortly after his arrival at McGill, Collip received what proved a historic "courtship call" from a charismatic middle-aged pharmacist named William McKenna. His checkbook in hand, the man identified himself as sales manager, trainer, promotional director, and chief contact man of a tiny upstart drug company incorporated in 1925 as Ayerst, McKenna, and Harrison, soon to be known as Ayerst Laboratories. The company boasted a paid-in capital of only $4,250. Nonetheless, the new corporation had just struck oil—cod liver oil—and McKenna, along with his four partners, all drug salesmen, had resigned their jobs and staked their futures on a plan to distribute Bottled Sunlight, an oil derived from Newfoundland codfish. They believed that patriotic Canadians were sure to prefer domestic fish oil over the available Norwegian brands. Perhaps they did, but the price differential was too enormous to swallow. Bottled Sunlight cost $1.50 per pint, while the imports from Norway were only 25¢.

The product on which Ayerst had pinned its hopes languished until McKenna had one of his bright ideas. He set up a display in a Toronto drugstore featuring healthy rats fed on the high-quality native cod liver oil versus puny rats fed on the "inferior" oil from Norway. The promotion, which attracted such crowds they had to call in the police, convinced the Canadian public that only Bottled Sunlight should be regulated and standardized—in other words, dubbed superior in every way. Snob appeal has been a hallmark of company strategy ever since (although it did backfire with the contraceptive Norplant in the 1990s); even Madeline Gray advised her 1950s readers that if they could swing it, ten cents a pill for Premarin, as compared to two cents for competing estrogens, was worth it.

It would have been interesting to have been a fly on the wall at Bill McKenna's initial meeting with Bert Collip. Ayerst Labs had no history. Only six months earlier, they'd been on the verge of closing shop. Their ice was preciously thin to attract a heavyweight like Collip. Why would an acknowledged genius accept support from so undercapitalized a crew when almost any of the great drug manufacturers—Lilly, Squibb, or Merck, to name only three—were eagerly scouting biochemists to help them develop new hormone products?

Among other reasons McKenna's pitch appealed to Collip was that Ayerst didn't yet have any in-house scientists on staff, nobody who'd visit and poke around, make interfering suggestions, and maybe try to take credit for Collip's original work. The scars from the insulin team inflicted seven years earlier came to dictate Collip's odd protocol now.

The first product to issue from the partnership of Ayerst Labs and Collip was called Emmenin, derived from the late-pregnancy urine of Canadian women. It was introduced in 1930 as the "first orally effective estrogen," but as a corporate history of the drug company explains, "Low activity, high cost, and problems of taste and odor lessened the chances for long-term survival of the product. Thus the laboratory embarked on a search for a new source."

Percheron stallions were the next source tried. Stallions are male, of course, but are said to have the most potent estrogen in their urine of any living animal of either gender. As the corporate history puts it, "The stallion urine showed a good degree of potency, although collection problems made dubious its potential as a sustained economic source."

Basically, the stallions kicked over the collection buckets.

The third source of urine proved to be the charm. The compliant mare, whose urine was "at least two and one half times [the potency] of human urine," carried the day and lent her name to the final product. The pitch to physicians by McKenna's sales force for this product that would make Ayerst's "first major impact on the pharmaceutical industry" went like this:

> Conjugated estrogens, developed exclusively by Ayerst, were extracted from mare's urine during the third to the tenth month of the eleven months pregnancy period, and blended across the seasons to produce a uniform mixture of sodium salts from the sulfate esters of the estrogenic substances.

Ayerst dubbed this Premarin. Doctors and pharmacists found the name (for *pre*gnant *mar*e's ur*in*e) apt and amusing, but we can only guess how many of the users understood what they were taking.

The name changes of Premarin's parent corporation may be confusing, so let us briefly trace the mergers and acquisitions that led to the dropping of the name Ayerst in 2002. The company that now owns Premarin is called simply Wyeth. In 1860, John Wyeth and his brother Frank opened a small drugstore on Walnut Street in Philadelphia. By the 1870s, they'd built an export trade to Canada, and in 1883 they opened a branch of their drugstore in Montreal. They had been there for forty-two years when Ayerst, McKenna, and Harrison was founded. A third company, American Home Products (AHP), was founded in 1926. Upon his death in 1929, Stuart Wyeth, son of John, left his controlling interest to his alma mater, Harvard University. In 1931, AHP bought Wyeth from Harvard. In 1943, AHP bought Ayerst as well. These two divisions of AHP, Wyeth and Ayerst, began a merger in 1987, which they completed in 1993, the year that Wyeth established the Women's Health Research Institute (a corporate front with goals for a health bureau). In 2002, AHP changed its name to Wyeth to "reflect its role as a global research-driven pharmaceutical company committed to solving the world's health problems through leading-edge biotechnology."

THE CHEMIST, HIS WIFE, AND HIS FÜHRER: SCHERING AND THE GERMAN GENIUS

Born in 1903 in Bremerhaven, Germany, Adolph Friedrich Johann Butenandt was eleven years younger than Bert Collip and lived a longer life. Collip died in 1965 at seventy-two, while Butenandt survived until 1995, harboring dark political secrets that are only beginning to emerge. Through an extraordinary decade, starting in 1928, these brilliant biochemists were going head-to-head in a high-stakes race to develop hormone products. Indeed, Schering, the German drug house, performed services for Butenandt identical to those Ayerst did for Collip. For example, Schering collected human pregnancy urine, from which Butenandt derived the raw materials for Progynon, essentially the same product as Collip's Emmenin and marketed to German women to treat hot flashes and night sweats. In a scenario similar to the Canadian one, Schering lost faith in the commercial prospects for human pregnancy urine (HPU) and soon switched to a mare's-urine product called Progynon2.

When the competition started, Collip was world famous, but Butenandt, barely out of graduate school, had the backing of a better established and richer pharmaceutical firm and the further advantage of a devoted collaborator, Erika von Ziegner, with whom, in 1929, he isolated the first sex hormone: folliculine (later identified as estrone).

Erika married Adolph in 1931, forsaking her own career to bear five daughters and two sons, although we know not what pillow talk of scientific matters may have continued through their marriage.

In contrast to Ayerst, the Montreal upstart, Butenandt's sponsor, founded in Berlin in 1851 by Ernst Schering, a dispensing chemist and distributor of fireworks, had grown into a mighty international corporation with thirty foreign subsidiaries and twenty manufacturing plants.

Schering knew it had a winner in Adolph. So whatever Adolph wanted, Adolph apparently got. Schering cut a deal with the Berlin police to make daily deliveries totaling 15,000 liters of men's urine, from which their star scientist isolated androstenedione in 1931 and testosterone in 1935. In 1934, he was first to identify progesterone in the female ovary. From the beginning, Butenandt also warned of the carcinogenic properties of some hormones under certain conditions because "they made cells divide."

Yet another Butenandt discovery led to the large-scale production of cortisone, and, in the 1950s, Butenandt was back in the science news when he coined the term *pheromone* for a substance secreted by an animal that affects the behavior of other animals of the same species. Unlike the retiring Collip, the German chemist loved popular acclaim, pomp and circumstance, and awards and honors. He collected medals from Germany, France, Sweden, and England, his favorite being the Grand Cross for Federal Services with Star. But in common with Collip, Butenandt found his path to the Nobel Prize in chemistry jinxed. Collip got a share of the money but not the honor. Butenandt got the honor without the money, as Hitler forbade him to leave Germany when he was named a laureate in 1939.

Not until ten years later did he make his way to Stockholm to collect his diploma and gold medal.

Apparently, Hitler didn't trust Butenandt, which I assumed to be a sign that he was no Nazi. But then I came across his obituary in the January 19, 1995, issue of *The Boston Globe*. It recalled that in 1935, Butenandt rejected a job offer from Harvard. That puzzled me. In the United States, we take it for granted that any non-Nazi scientist who had a chance to exit

Germany in the Hitler era did. A little math: Adolph Butenandt was thirty-two years old. Hitler was growing more aggressive and bent on war. Adolph was the father of small children. How could he turn down Harvard if he didn't have some regard for his führer after all?

I needed to raise the question of Butenandt's politics with someone in the know. The natural choice was Carl Djerassi, who was born in Vienna in 1923 and became the youngest of the extraordinary cohort of sex-hormone scientists preceding and following World War II whose research laid the groundwork for practically all the products we use today. Djerassi is the father of the modern progestins in oral contraceptives and calls himself "the mother of the pill."

Carl Djerassi e-mailed me right back. "Butenandt was not the most pleasant of men but a first-class chemist," he said. "He was one of the most famous steroid chemists of all times and certainly a Nazi, although not of the really vicious kind. Perhaps one might call him the Heisenberg of chemistry," a reference to the 1932 German Nobelist in physics.

Recent scholarship by scientists and educators such as Benno Muller-Hill, a professor of genetics at the University of Cologne, and Robert Proctor, an American historian and author of *The Nazi War on Cancer*, has unveiled some of Butenandt's Nazi sympathies. For example, Proctor discovered a 1941 radio interview in which Butenandt praised Hitler: "Of course! There is a great deal being done for cancer research in Germany. In every part of the Reich there are magnificent institutes for which the führer has provided large sums of money."

In any event, Harvard was outbid; Butenandt was persuaded to stay in Germany by the drug industry and the government. Schering, for example, increased his compensation, paying him 160,000 reichsmarks (which would approximate $1 million today) for his patents on Progynon.

The German chemical industry guaranteed Butenandt's well-being, and in 1936, at age thirty-two, he got a prestigious job—director of Berlin's Kaiser Wilhelm Institute for Biochemistry (later renamed the Max Planck Society), which might be compared to being appointed a director of the National Institutes of Health in the United States. According to Proctor, Butenandt always had the newest and largest equipment in his lab, received funds from the Nazi regime, and never distanced himself from the Nazis. His research was classified as important to the war and "his people" were not sent to the front. (His two horses also got special treatment: They were saved from slaughter.) During the war, Adolph and Erika were reported to have maintained a "civilized life that included classical music, skating, tennis, and table tennis." They were religious enough to say grace at every meal, and described as "patriotic but not fanatic."

Butenandt was not anti-Semitic: He saved two Jewish scientists from death—Carl Neuberg, whom he helped set up an underground laboratory in Berlin, and Alfred Gottschalk. In later years, when the question of Nazi sympathies was raised, some Jews spoke kindly of Butenandt, though he never openly defended them. In the postwar era, he was described as a "one-person de-Nazification whitewasher" who "helped a lot of former colleagues under attack to clear themselves," maintaining that they were "pure scientists studying facts outside of moral judgments," as Proctor describes it. Yet Butenandt pulled out every stop to prevent Otmar Frieherr von Verschur, a eugenicist and director of the Third Reich Institute for Hereditary Biology and Purity who wrote a famous textbook on "racial cleansing," from being tried as a Nazi criminal. Then, in 1984, *Murderous Science*, an exposé by genetics professor Benno Muller-Hill, revealed that von Verschur was, in fact, an administrator of horrific Auschwitz experiments and the boss of the notorious Dr. Joseph Mengele.

HIGH CRIMES OR MISDEMEANORS?

In the fall of 1944, as defeat was near, Butenandt moved to Tubingen to get out of the way of the invading Allied forces. He directed Dr. Gunther Hillman, his closest associate, to destroy all documents marked "Secret Matters of State." Later, Butenandt denied that the Kaiser Wilhelm Institute was ever involved in euthanasia programs. I believe him. After all, he himself never had to go near Auschwitz; he had only to study hormone levels in the blood and urine of its prisoners. However, as Alison Abbott of *Nature* magazine concludes, "It seems that Butenandt cleaned out any incriminating letters from his files—if there had been any. We are only left with deduction, and knowing of his character, it seems unlikely that Butenandt was unaware of what was going on in his institute. Why he would have turned a blind eye is not known."

I'll tell you why: I believe Butenandt was motivated to turn that "blind eye" in order to pay back Schering for having sponsored his career. He wanted to help the company maintain its leadership in the hormone lines, and most specifically he wanted to help his patron establish an effective dose of the drug ethinyl estradiol so that it could be used *safely* as a contraceptive. And he would not have to go anywhere near Auschwitz to do it—just poke around with the blood samples the Nazis sent him.

Besides Butenandt's profound gratitude to Schering for its patronage from his youth onward—a patronage that allowed him to become a Nobelist before the age of forty—he also had the opportunity to make a great contribution to the applied use of hormones, because he had access to a captive group of women for his trials. So he had both motive and opportunity to commit his crime. And make no mistake about it: However much he had convinced himself that his intentions were for the greater good, his research on death-camp inmates was nonetheless a huge and horrible crime.

I can only add that, after the war, if von Verschur and others had been interrogated, the trail could have led to Butenandt. Thus, he who protected Jewish colleagues in the 1930s went on to protect their persecutors ten years later. But I strongly believe that his abiding loyalty throughout the war was not to Hitler but to Schering, his patron.

BIRTH CONTROL AND THE MASTER RACE

Should you ever visit the Schering Museum, in the oldest school building in the Berlin-Wedding district, you may get to see the first patient leaflets on hormones, prepared for the public in 1934 and introducing three new products, all derived from Butenandt's original work. These included Progynon, an estrogen; Proluton, a progesterone; and Testoviron, a.k.a. Proviron, the male sex hormone. These leaflets attempt to describe the effects of these previously unknown, highly active substances to an astonished citizenry. By 1938, again based on Butenandt's discoveries, Schering scientists Hans Herloff Inhoffen and Walter Hohlweg synthesized the aforementioned ethinyl estradiol, which remains the most popular estrogen used in birth control pills to this day.

In 1943, on the night of November 22, a bombing raid destroyed Schering's main administration building, the "redbrick palace" on the Muellerstrasse. Important research work, records, and drug manufacturing processes went up in flames, but it didn't halt Schering's hormone research, which now focused on "the inhibition of ovulation with progesterone in women" and was deemed a success in 1944.

You may wonder why research on hormones for birth control was continued during the darkest days of World War II. What did worry-free sex have to do with the war effort? But this was Hitler's Germany, where eugenics and ethnic cleansing were primary goals, making sterilization and contraception high priorities toward the achievement of an Aryan master race. A once-classified Nuremberg document states that "greenhouses were built at Auschwitz to grow a rare South American plant from which female hormones could be made to lead to sterilization of persons without their knowledge."

In the mid-1950s, numerous Auschwitz survivors told Dr. Jean Jofen, a psychologist at City University in New York, that they were fed daily doses of liquid estrogen in their rutabaga soup. The women stopped menstruating and the men lost their sex drive, just as the Nazis expected. But these refugees were not left permanently sterile. Indeed, Dr. Jofen, herself born in Vienna, had occasion to question these Auschwitz survivors because she was testing the IQs of their five-year-old children at a Hebrew parochial school.

When I interviewed Dr. Jofen in 1976, she recalled that "the synthetic estrogens were similar to those found in the current pill. They just poured it in the soup. There was no dosage." She later said the contraceptive was called salitrum. There were long-term repercussions to this fortified soup. In a paper presented at the fifth World Congress of Jewish Studies in Jerusalem, Jofen reported that after testing hundreds of children of holocaust survivors, the Auschwitz contingent had the lowest IQ range. Jofen wondered if the hormone experiments did some permanent harm to the ova of these mothers. The comparison group, mothers who'd been interned at other concentration camps, also endured dreadful conditions, but they received no estrogen and their children's IQs were higher.

Any scientist who discovers a new drug is curious to know how it will finally play out in humans. But humans aren't laboratory animals, as many scientists have lamented. How do you get them to take the drug at the same time every day? How do you make sure that they stay on it, and how do you convince them to let you draw their blood? Throughout the 1950s, these same questions would plague Gregory Pincus and John Rock as well as their patron, Katharine McCormick, heiress to a farm-machinery fortune, as they searched for suitable subjects for their trials on the first U.S. birth control pill. At times it seemed hopeless, as McCormick's correspondence with Margaret Sanger reveals. One problem was that the scientists lived in Massachusetts, where birth control research was a crime punishable by imprisonment. Rock did his preliminary clinical work in the guise of treating menstrual disorders, and Pincus supervised some small trials in Worcester State Psychiatric Hospital (on men as well as women), but none of this work was adequate for drug acceptance by the FDA.

The year 1953 found McCormick complaining to Sanger:

> Human females are not as easy to investigate as are rabbits in cages. The latter can be intensively controlled all the time, whereas the human females leave town at unexpected times and so cannot be examined at a certain period. [T]hey also forget to take the medicine sometimes—in which case the whole experiment has to begin over again—for scientific accuracy must be maintained or the resulting data are worthless.

By 1955, McCormick was so frustrated and discouraged that some of her postings to Sanger sounded loony: "[We need] a cage of ovulating females to experiment with."

The following year Pincus—like Butenandt before him—found his "cage of ovulating females" at a new housing project, part of a slum-clearance program in Río Piedras, a suburb of San Juan, Puerto Rico. The "ovulating females," the poorest of the poor, had no place else to go, and, short of sterilization, no other birth control options. Dr. Edris Rice-Wray, medical director of the Puerto Rican Family Planning Association, was placed in charge. A colleague at the medical school pressed female medical students to join the trials, but they wouldn't stick to it, due to nausea, dizziness, headaches, and vomiting, even though they were threatened with lower grades for quitting.

The Río Piedras women got the same experimental doses, but they had fewer alternatives than the medical students. Many dropped out, but they were replaced, for as social worker Iris Rodriguez wrote: "We have more cases than what we can take for our study." Indeed, it was true that thousands of women tried Enovid, the first birth control pill approved for contraception in the United States in 1960. I was there. I heard all about the thoroughness of the studies from the manufacturer and the FDA. I was there again in 1963 when Senator Hubert Humphrey, investigating the Food and Drug Administration, discovered that in fact only 132 women out of thousands had the stamina to stay on Enovid for a year or longer. No wonder it called for superhuman determination to stick with the regimen: The dosages were ten times higher than they are today.

Others independently came up with some of the same findings reported by Butenandt, and at around the same time. James Bertram Collip in Canada and Edward Doisy in the United States made similar estrogen discoveries, while Leopold Ruzicka (a Czech scientist) did near-identical work on testosterone. But no one else accomplished so much in that one decade, and the pinnacle, Schering's contraceptive estrogen, has certainly passed the unforgiving test of time. Butenandt was Schering's star and beloved genius, the founder of their great sex-hormone line, the estrogens, the progesterone, and even the testosterone. There cannot be doubt that he retained access to the earlier hormones that came directly from his lab, or even to those of the next generation, including the excellent ethinyl estradiol, seventeen times stronger than the estradiol produced by our bodies and readily available by mouth. That Schering creation alone—approved for use in humans in 1949—is a component in nine out of ten twenty-first-century birth control pills.

CATASTROPHE AT THE CHARITE

However, the initial plans Schering had for ethinyl estradiol were put on ice, and kept there for a dozen years, when England's *Nature* magazine published the formula for a competing oral estrogen that was not only cheaper but also in the public domain. Moreover—and perhaps more to the point—the clinical trials of Schering's drug at Berlin's Charite Hospital had met with disaster . . . a disaster of such magnitude that even in Nazi Germany, doctors wanted nothing more to do with ethinyl estradiol. As recalled by Schering pharmacologist Karl Junkmann, "It was overdosed by a factor of several hundred percent. It resulted in almost uncontrollable bleeding."

THE PANDORA'S BOX OF SIR CHARLIE DODDS, OR CHARLIE TRUMPS "THE DEVIL'S CHEMISTS" AND HAS HELL TO PAY

But if we fail, then the whole world will sink into the abyss of a new dark age made more sinister, and perhaps more protracted, by the lights of perverted science. Let us therefore brace ourselves to our duties, and so bear ourselves that if the British Empire and its

Commonwealth last for a thousand years, men will still say: "This
was their finest hour."

— WINSTON CHURCHILL

In 1938, the opening year of the greatest experiment ever performed
on women, Winston Churchill was out on a limb in England, warning his
countrymen that Hitler intended war. Few paid attention, even though the
führer already held Austria and was poised to take Czechoslovakia. Recovering from the trauma of World War I, struggling to come out of an economic depression, the British weren't in a mood to hear Churchill's
message, preferring instead to support Prime Minister Neville Chamber-
lain's doomed appeasement policies.

There were exceptions, of course, among them a tiny corps of distinguished chemists, including Edward Charles Dodds, director of the Courtauld Institute of Biochemistry at Middlesex Hospital in London and the
father of diethylstilbestrol or DES, the first synthetic estrogen to make a
huge commercial splash the world over. Affable and kindly, a regular at
international chemistry events, Charles Dodds frequently received ominous news from Germany. He was often reminded that German chemistry, dangerously ahead of Britain's on many frontiers, was being
conscripted in the service of Hitler's most evil fantasies. Dodds often discussed his fears and worries with his eminent colleague and friend Dr.
Robert Robinson, director of the Dyson Perrins Laboratory at Oxford University. They pooled their information and passed it on to Churchill, providing the background for the future prime minister to cry out against the
"perverted science" of the Third Reich. As Dodds and Robinson were
doing research in sex hormones, they were particularly interested in Butenandt's work and in the uses Schering made of it. They were concerned

that Schering had major ties to I. G. Farben, a German cartel of five large corporations that dealt with all sorts of chemicals, including poison gases and rocket fuels, and which, drawn by free labor to the death camps, would soon build an industrial complex at Auschwitz for the production of synthetic rubber and oil.

At war's end, General Dwight D. Eisenhower assigned a team of civilian and military experts to make an exhaustive investigation of Farben's contribution to the Nazi effort. When members of Germany's industrial elite were tried at Nuremberg, the key role that chemistry had played in the Third Reich was underlined by the name applied to these criminals: "the Devil's Chemists."

The Devil's Chemist Dodds feared most was Butenandt. Perhaps he and Robinson were a little bit envious, for no other steroid chemist in the world had such achievements to his credit. On the other hand, these Englishmen were not engaged in heads-on professional competition, for they were on a different track, trying to develop what are called nonsteroidal estrogens, in contrast to Butenandt's, which were steroidal.

The nonsteroidal estrogen is simpler. It lacks the four interlocking carbon rings that characterize the natural steroidal hormones and their derivatives. Dodds and Robinson, working separately, were aiming for a simpler compound—a compound without the rings of carbon, completely synthetic, unrelated to any natural substance, strong enough to take by mouth, stable, and very inexpensive. And oh yes—it would have to deliver all the same benefits as existing steroidal estrogens.

Dodds had been working hard on this since 1934 and was almost there, but one or two final mysteries remained for him to unlock, a term he often used to convey the challenges of chemistry.

Some time around New Year's Day 1938, Dodds and Robinson called a hasty meeting to discuss the latest rumor from Berlin. Schering had applied for a patent on estradiol. Dodds and Robinson agreed this was absurd and unethical. Estradiol is not a patentable substance. Estrogen molecules belong to nature. They belong to God. They belong to— women.

Dodds wondered if Butenandt held the ethinyl estradiol patent. He didn't. The patent named two in-house scientists in Schering's Berlin Hormone Research Department, Walter Hohlweg and Hans Herloff Inhoffen.

Inhoffen, a brilliant chemistry student from Hanover, Germany, studied in England in the late 1920s "to get to know the land and the people." In 1935, according to a history of the development of ethinyl estradiol, "Schering made it possible for Inhoffen to spend time in England until 1936. During that time, he worked at the Courtauld Institute of Biochemistry in London as an assistant to Charles Dodds. The group working with Dodds was concerned at the time with investigations of nonsteroidal estrogenically active substances called stilbenes. These investigations that were to lead in 1938 to the preparation of stilbestrol . . . were naturally of great interest to Schering as hormone manufacturers. In 1936 Inhoffen returned to Berlin and worked until 1945 as department manager in Schering's main laboratory."

Dodds must have been beside himself. Was Schering now preparing to patent some form of the nonsteroidal estrogen that Dodds had pursued for so long? Was his ex-assistant, Inhoffen, a Nazi spy? (Some sixty years later, in 1999, on receiving an "Inhoffen Medal" from the Technical University in Braunschweig, Carl Djerassi would also wonder. "It was a rather obvious question," he writes, "for someone with my paranoia-inducing background as a Hitler refugee." Turns out that, like Butenandt, Inhoffen was a Nazi considered "more or less clean. . . . I would say," Djerassi's informant explained, "that Inhoffen was what is known in this country to be 'ein kleiner Nazi'" (a little Nazi).

"Such products must stay in the public domain," Dodds insisted, referrring to synthetic estrogen. "Those Germans are trying to corner the entire field of sex hormones, and use the profits to fund Hitler," Robinson added. They were told that estradiol might be used as a weapon, but they didn't know for what. Would this be a means to Hitler's "final solution" to sterilize and eliminate Jews, Gypsies, cripples, and maybe the British one day?

After a while, as if they were mischievous schoolboys, they concocted an audacious plan to give Butenandt, Inhoffen, Schering, and their boss Hitler a big black eye.

Robinson's nonsteroidal research was at an earlier stage than Dodds's, but he had some excellent ideas and offered to help cheer Dodds to the finish line. They would pool their resources. Their labs would work together. Maybe some of their countrymen didn't know it, but this was war. For a suitable crash effort, they would enlist all workers at both facilities, even the undergraduate students. Dodds could keep the principal credit, but Robinson and his people would give their all—for Dodds, for the King, for England. Schering was about to make a killing with its patented ethinyl estradiol. If Dodds and Robinson hurried, they might stop the private ownership of estrogen molecules in its tracks.

Very soon thereafter, Wilfred Lawson, a chemist on Dodds's staff, scribbled a new formulation on the back of an envelope. Leon Golberg, an Oxford student of Robinson's, performed the actual synthesis of diethylstilbestrol by heating one gram of a similar substance to 205°C. All at once, it was done. The formula worked. Dodds rushed the experiment into publication in the form of a fifteen-paragraph article in the magazine *Nature* on February 15, 1938.

This would give the world a cheap and powerful estrogen everyone could use. Any of Schering's hopes for a big export business in estradiol were dashed, along with plans to control the world's hormone markets. The estrogen diethylstilbestrol could be taken in liquid form or as a pill and—a sensational bargain—would cost only $2 a gram, compared to estradiol's $300. It came to be known as DES in the United States and stilbestrol in England.

DES was a novel and daring product, constructed entirely from a chemical base. It produced the same feminizing effects as estrogens derived from animals and plants but was three times more powerful. Anyone could make it, because in publishing his formula Dodds threw away his own patent rights. It was wartime, and he did it to checkmate Adolph Butenandt and Adolf Hitler, not to encourage experimentation on women, though he began to entertain regrets almost at once. A daring inventor, Dodds was at the same time a very conservative physician. He stood in awe of the female reproductive system, which, as he often explained, was but partly understood. Here is a statement from him that I have quoted over the years:

"We should always be humbled when we think of what we do not know about the female reproductive cycle. We still have no understanding of the mechanism that makes one Graafian follicle in one of the ovaries of a normal woman maturate and ovulate each month. This is a baffling problem. Until we know that mechanism that selects one Graafian follicle, out of perhaps hundreds of thousands, to maturate each month, we still have to proceed with caution on any long-term hormonal treatment of the human female."

Dodds had no thought whatever that his stilbestrol would be given to healthy women. I asked him what he had thought it would be used for. "Estrogen deficiency," he replied. I asked, "Are you using the term the way gynecologists call menopause an 'estrogen deficiency disease'?"

"Oh, no," he responded. "Not for a natural menopause, but maybe for a while if a woman has had her ovaries taken out. We don't cut out healthy ovaries here in England so much, but in your country they have a fad for it.

"Do you want to know what I was thinking at the moment I realized we succeeded? I was grateful that stilbestrol would do all the things that estrogen can do, and more reliably and in a price range that most people could afford. I wished we had found it three years earlier. I was thinking of a beautiful child named Jessica, whom I tried to treat with estrogen injections in 1935. She was born minus her ovaries, and when she was thirteen years old her mother brought her to me to ask if I could do something to help her become a 'normal' young woman, develop breasts and so on. Well, I tried. I gave her a series of estrogen injections that were painful and expensive and didn't really work. It started to look as though they would, but then they didn't. The estrogen source was unpredictable and too weak. Jessica and her family were unbearably sad. If you take too much stilbestrol or take it for too long, you may get cancer. It stimulates cells to grow faster, which is not always a good idea. But in rare cases, if you really need it, it's a miracle—like insulin."

Dodds was always against the automatic prescribing of estrogen for any reason. He was sickened when he heard about the work of Dr. Karl John Karnaky in Houston, the first to use DES widely to "prevent miscarriages." Dodds sent Karnaky a study that he himself had performed, showing that in rabbits and rats, the drug *caused* miscarriages. That never stopped Karnaky, who as an old man boasted that he had given DES to 150,000 women.

In the months right after he synthesized stilbestrol, Dodds was already fretting about a cancer link. On occasion, stilbestrol powder blew around in his lab, and he noticed that the men on his staff who handled it, their suspenders puffing out over their shirts, were growing breasts. This suggested to him that stilbestrol might cause breast cancer in men. Dodds rushed out samples, meticulously packaged, to a young researcher at the National Cancer Institute just being established in the United States. The researcher, Dr. Michael Boris Shimkin, was thorough, precise, outspoken, and fearless. By the time he died in 1989, many had come to consider him the greatest cancer researcher of his era. He was one of the first to question the value of radical mastectomies and to challenge the American Medical Association for its ties to the tobacco industry. Dodds asked Shimkin to investigate the carcinogenicity of stilbestrol in male rodents. In the October 1940 issue of *The Journal of the National Cancer Institute*, Shimkin, in collaboration with Hugh Grady, reported that stilbestrol produced breast cancers in both male and female mice of a certain strain. The females were bred to develop cancer spontaneously, but not so the male mice. Shimkin informed Dodds that cancer in the males was a testimony to the power of diethylstilbestrol.

At Dodds's request, Shimkin tried to inform Americans why Dodds, the father of DES, did not want it to be casually employed—at least not until many more studies were performed. Many in the U.S. cancer research community heard the message and took it to heart. Few civilians knew it, but the top animal toxicology and cancer experts were trying to dissuade the Food and Drug Administration (FDA) from giving the green light to Dodds's brainchild.

The Shimkin-Grady paper was far from the only warning about DES. Dr. Charles Geschicter of Johns Hopkins reported in *Radiology* magazine that he produced mammary cancer in Wistar rats by injecting them with DES and other estrogens. Probably more shocking was the much later discovery by Dr. Karnaky of Houston and Drs. George and Olive Smith of Harvard and others who followed their lead of the abnormalities in the reproductive organs of children of mothers given DES in pregnancy.

But even earlier, in 1939 and '40, in *The American Journal of Anatomy* and other publications, J. R. R. Greene, V. W. Burrill, and A. C. Ivy published a series of articles on what they termed "experimental intersexuality," showing the impact on animal fetuses whose mothers were treated in pregnancy with estrogens, including DES. Female rat offspring had enlarged uteruses and structural changes in the vagina and ovaries. Males had small and improperly developed penises and changes in other sexual and reproductive organs.

In 1976, after discovery of the tragedies in some DES offspring, the rare cancers in daughters, the increased rate of testicular cancers in sons, the anatomical abnormalities afflicting both sexes, I asked the Smiths if they had been aware of any of this research. Dr. Olive Smith stated, "Before we even started any clinical work at all we went through all the literature."

"However," her husband said, "you can do all kinds of things to rats and mice by giving them overdoses." This scientific shrug of the shoulders cannot reassure the maimed.

At that point, I wished that Dodds were still alive so I could tell him about this bizarre conversation, but then again, maybe not. "It wasn't your fault, Charlie," I said to myself as I collected my tape recorder and left. "You did everything you could to stop it."

And so did Shimkin, who as it happened was assigned by the U.S. Army Medical Corps as a public health doctor in Germany in 1944–45, giving aid to concentration camp survivors and documenting the condition of their health. He would explain the DES story this way to anyone who would listen:

Charlie Dodds would not have published so precipitously, he wouldn't have necessarily sped his formula around the globe, but he saw this as the one thing he could do to help stop Hitler. He had great anger at the German scientists trying to corner the market on female sex hormones on behalf of the German pharmaceutical combines. His main motivation was to synthesize a powerful, inexpensive estrogen that would stay in the public domain. He was outraged at the patenting of molecules of estrogen by the German firms. He was driven to provide something that the general public could get cheaper, and that still would be available when war came.

Born in 1899, Dodds lived to seventy-three. When I knew him in the 1960s, he was about five foot seven, stocky, bald on top, and wore horn-rimmed glasses. The son of a shoe salesman who had known hard times, he loved good wines and his Rolls-Royce. Compared to the productive Butenandt, he may have been only an A– as a biochemist, but as a human being he was A+.

In 1963, I got the professional break of my life—an interview with Dodds. I was writing on women's health for several magazines, and this often meant reporting on the pill, the biggest women's medical news of that decade and perhaps the century. Because of my aunt Sally, I myself didn't take it, but for other women, those lacking a near relative who'd died young from an estrogen-dependent cancer, I held an open mind. Certainly the press releases I received from Planned Parenthood, as well as from the manufacturers, had nothing but good to say.

However, every time I wrote on the pill, I received an unusual volume of reader mail focusing on side effects that their doctors had not prepared them for or taken seriously when they occurred. A litany of similar statements cropped up: "I was up against a stone wall . . . a brick wall, a wall of indifference." "He told me it was all in my head." "He said don't worry your pretty little head about it." "He said, 'My wife takes it; would I give her anything that would harm her?'"

Many a doctor was reported to have told patients that their complaints were psychogenic, due to their fear of sexual freedom.

The readers, however, knew exactly what the side effects were, ranging from the top of their heads (headache, hair loss, stroke) all the way down to their formerly healthy young ankles and feet (swelling, blood clots). The attitudes of these doctors were anathema to me. I desperately needed guidance, a real expert who would be candid with me so that I could pass reliable information on to my readers.

One day, at the Academy of Medicine Library in New York, I came across the text of a speech by Charles Dodds, then the president of the Royal College of Physicians, exhorting doctors to be wary of the pill. The reasons he gave—the metabolism, the ovaries, the potential infertility and cancer and birth defects—astonished me, but he described them in a way that made perfect sense. Hormones were good to cure diseases, he said, but were dangerous for longtime use in healthy people. And then I read his biography. This was the man who'd discovered the first synthetic estrogen. Here was the equivalent of Einstein, the physicist who'd opposed the nuclear weapons race. Not only that, Dodds announced he would use his pulpit to warn doctors and women against "promiscuous" use of the pill.

I wrote to him, even sent him some reader mail. Could this symptom be from the pill, could that? Depression . . . loss of sex drive . . . weight gain . . . jaundice . . . skin blotches . . . bleeding gums . . . urinary infections. And Dodds explained the medical reasons behind the complaints. For example, he said that hormones were among the most powerful of drugs, serving a broad, not a narrow, function, and they could alter the metabolism in every cell and organ of the body. The depression, in his view, was less likely to be from "fear of carefree sex" so much as from depletion in B vitamins—folic acid among others—the lack of which could alter brain chemistry enough to cause feelings of sadness and despondency.

The post-pill infertility, the failure to get back normal menstrual cycles for quite a long time, came because the pill interrupted the "normal dance" of the pituitary and ovaries. Dodds thought it was wrong to start a woman on fertility drugs instead of first suggesting a healthy diet.

I could hardly believe that a scientist of Dodds's stature could find the time to brief me on the physiology of the pill, to take my phone calls, to send me papers he wrote and speeches he gave, but he did. He also warned that the dosages in the pills appeared to be inexcusably higher than was needed to do the job. He suggested that a tenth of the original doses might be enough. He turned out to be right on target.

Dodds was widely called upon to consult with industry on drug safety and additives to food. He approved the use of DES as a growth stimulant in animals, but only if the pellets implanted in the head and neck of animals were removed a week (at minimum) before slaughter, so the drug would not still be in the animal when it entered the food chain.

As a patriot and as a scientist (if far less so in his role as a physician), Dodds remained proud of his discovery. When he was knighted and became Sir Edward Charles Dodds in 1964, a stained-glass window to honor him was placed in an ancient building called the Hall of the Worshipful Society of the Apothecaries of London. The heraldic crest displays a woman in a blue off-the-shoulder dress holding an open book showing the chemical formula for diethylstilbestrol, the point being to remind posterity that this compound was "as available as an open book to anyone who wanted it" and had never been patented. Dodds loved to live well, and he could have made a fortune from DES royalties, far more than the mere million dollars Butenandt earned on Progynon.

FOOTNOTE TO HISTORY #1

During the war, Dodds and Butenandt, to no one's surprise, had a falling out, but in postwar years they got back on speaking terms and had many a discussion about their mutual concerns for estrogens and cancer.

Eventually, in a bizarre twist, the Nobel Prize for a DES application (this one in the physiology of medicine, in 1966) went to Dr. Charles Brenton Huggins, a Chicago urologist who used the drug to treat prostate cancer in men. The idea was that "by depriving cancer cells of the correct signals, the growth of tumors could be slowed down, at least temporarily." To my mind, Huggins was heartless. He described the tragic condition of the DES families as "a put-up job to cheat Lilly out of millions of dollars."

Gullibility and wishful thinking on female hormones, for one purpose or another, have, alas, never ceased. Consider the extreme life-extension benefits claimed for hormone treatments in aging women, which again rose to dangerous levels in the 1990s, as they had in the 1960s, before receding for a time. I began to wonder if it was the doctors, not the patients, who might need head exams.

COMING TO AMERICA: COMMUNITY INTEREST OF THE U.S. DRUG INDUSTRY

As soon as Dodds's formula appeared in *Nature*, free to copy by all comers, a plethora of American drug companies, most notably Eli Lilly and Squibb, but also Abbott Laboratories, Sharp & Dohme, and Upjohn, were distributing samples to doctors and seeking instructions from the FDA on how to get approval. Lilly launched its own research program, under the direction of Dr. Don Carlos Hines, while Squibb's Dr. Sidney Newcomer called on interested physicians, including Karnaky, encouraging them to do research that Squibb would help them prepare for publication.

But alarm bells were ringing, and it wasn't just DES that set them off. Dodds's estrogen was the newest addition to a family of drugs already indicted for causing cancer. Back in 1932, Antoine Lacassagne, who would one day win the coveted UN Prize for Cancer Research, gave Butenandt's estrogens to mice and induced mammary cancer. By the end of the 1930s, Shimkin, Dodds, and anyone else who wanted to check this out at a medical library would have been quite startled at the sheer weight of the warnings already published in prestigious journals. Furthermore, on rumors that requests to market DES were pouring into the FDA, the *Journal of the American Medical Association* (*JAMA*) published a powerful editorial against the drug on December 23, 1939, titled "Estrogen Therapy—A Warning":

"Regarding conflicting reports about DES . . . a thorough investigation of this compound is in order before it can be prescribed for routine therapy. . . . The possibility of carcinoma cannot be ignored . . . it appears likely that the medical profession may be importuned to prescribe to patients large doses of high potency estrogens, such as stilbestrol, because of the ease of administration of these products."

In that same issue, the Council on Pharmacy and Chemistry (which included George N. Papanicolaou, originator of the Pap smear) cautioned that "because the product is so potent and because the possibility of harm must be recognized, the Council is of the opinion that it should not be recognized for general use at the present time . . . and that its use by the general medical profession should not be undertaken until further studies have led to a better understanding of the functions of the drug."

Nonetheless, by the end of 1940, a dozen drug companies had asked the FDA for approval to market diethylstilbestrol. The agency made it known that it would turn down any application but that the companies had the right to protest, fearing that if the press got wind of the situation, it would bring the cancer fears to public attention. The manufacturers, rather than fighting the decision, met together and decided to withdraw their applications, and to regroup.

The regrouping that followed was a first blueprint for joint spin doctoring by the drug companies and it laid down the basis for the formation of Big Pharma, the powerful industry lobby that would officially start business in 1951. Meanwhile, under tight discipline, the companies agreed to pool their resources to construct a "master file" on DES. Four companies, which became known as the Small Committee, would do the lion's share of the work. Lilly's Don Carlos Hines was the head of the group. Winthrop and Upjohn were members, and Dr. J. A. Morrell of Squibb contributed a most impressive collection of articles. (Impressive, that is, to the FDA perhaps, but it horrified Dodds, who recalled the dreaded "master file" to me with bitter emotion twenty-five years later.) That file contained 257 articles on the successful use of DES.

There were two divisions in the DES army. The drug-company doctors, Hines and Morrell, led the first; the second was headed by a dynamic Washington lobbyist-publicist, Carson P. Frailey, the executive vice president of a trade group, the American Drug Manufacturers Association.

Frailey's campaign opened on January 28, 1941, when he was host to a meeting at the Washington Hotel. He explained his scheme to round up doctors across the country and enlist them to write to the FDA. Fifty-four doctors cooperated, describing their experiences with more than 5,000 patients. Only four doctors felt that DES should not be approved.

By May 12, Frailey announced a nearly done deal. He sent a letter to the Small Committee with good news: "The time now seems propitious to suggest that you re-file your new drug application for stilbestrol. I am making no commitments that the application will be permitted to become effective, but the suggestion offered has official background."

The drug-company physicians understood from the letter that someone in power at the FDA was on their side of the battle. On September 19, 1941, the fall of the Japanese attack on Pearl Harbor, the FDA officially

WITHDRAWN

CHAPTER 3

How Has Premarin Fared in the United States, and Who Was Robert Wilson?

Bill McKenna was "an enthusiastic man, a man with a vision," according to the corporate history of Ayerst Labs. "Unusually attuned to the trends of his industry," he established a subsidiary in Rouses Point, New York, in 1934, was elected chairman, and "served in an unofficial capacity as Ayerst's ambassador to both the United States and Canadian governments. He represented his company in discussion of such delicate matters as food and drug legislation, and tariffs."

McKenna lived until 1958, long enough to establish Premarin as the number one menopause treatment in North America. Indeed, Premarin soon was to estrogen as Kleenex was to disposable hanky. As McKenna rose from rank-and-file to riches, he acknowledged his gratitude to Dr. James Bertram Collip and his pride that such a great man looked upon him as a friend. Nor did McKenna conceal his debt to Carson P. Frailey, the lobbyist who'd shown him how to run circles around the FDA. McKenna's behind-the-scenes participation in the DES campaign was the best dress rehearsal for trying to launch a new drug that anyone could hope for. In later years, McKenna would tell his staff, "Frailey figured out how the FDA *really* works." Under Frailey's tutelage, McKenna understood the drill, knew how to identify allies in the agency and how to make sure the papers he sent in landed on the right desks. He also learned how to obfuscate the cancer connection, although tumors of the breast, cervix, endometrium, pituitary, testicles, kidney, and bone marrow were associated with estrogen, including Premarin, in mice, rats, rabbits, hamsters, and dogs. However, McKenna never believed that he was in the business of giving cancer to women. Like others, he succumbed to denial and wishful thinking on the relevance of "overdoses" in small animals. Yet by the time he submitted his papers to the FDA, several years after Premarin came onto the Canadian market but still early in the Premarin time line, he *had* to know about the ubiquitous endometrial disturbances in humans.

Here are the facts: Nature gives the uterus a rapid response to hormone stimulation so that it can "hit the ground running," as it were, when a fertilized egg comes looking for a home. After the first year on Premarin, one woman in ten already has potentially malignant overgrowths in the lining of her uterus. By the third year, the number rises to one in three, and continues to climb thereafter. If left untreated, one in five long-term Premarin users has a lifetime chance of developing endometrial cancer, whereas for nonusers the chance is one in fifty. Nonetheless, on May 8, 1942, McKenna received approval to market Premarin in the United States.

On McKenna's watch, the Premarin ads were charming, like the man himself. Designed to foster fantasies of a fountain of youth, they featured glamorous women of a certain age having fun, being admired, sometimes waltzing with impeccably dressed handsome gentlemen who (you could tell) adored them. In the hallowed tradition of McKenna's Newfoundland Cod Liver Oil coup, the ads were distinctly upscale, which made sense, since the price for Premarin was five times higher than competing DES products, ten cents a pill in contrast to two. At rival companies, which were rapidly losing sales on their bargain DES to Premarin, anger, envy, and dismay erupted when the meaning of Premarin's name and featured ingredient dawned on them. But at one firm, Parke-Davis, there was mirth. That was because their iconoclastic president, Harry Loynd, who, like McKenna, had begun as a humble salesman, was contemptuous of both doctors and drugs. His motto was "drugs are to sell, not to take," and he viewed doctors as the most "gullible" of men. "Indeed," he had often proclaimed to his staff, "if we put horse manure in a capsule we could sell it to 95 percent of those doctors."

TAME THE DIRTY OLD SAVAGE BEAST

After McKenna retired, the ads for Premarin took an ugly, nasty, and misogynistic turn, featuring repulsive, witchlike women, angry or depressed, hapless-looking fixtures in their doctors' waiting rooms, menacing their children, or nagging or humiliating their husbands. A medical journal ad in 1977 depicts a harpy who obviously has just done something awful, possibly hit her teenaged son in the mouth, for his hand covers the lower part of his face and he appears in pain. He, his sister, and his father are glaring at the harpy with loathing and fear. Father is comforting the sister, who might be about to cry, and he is clutching his *unfinished* newspaper. The harpy has interrupted the tranquility of the family home. The Premarin copy states: "Almost any tranquilizer might calm her down . . . but at her age estrogen might be what she really needs. Patients taking Premarin alone often report relief of emotional symptoms due to estrogen deficiency . . . and an improved sense of well-being."

Other ads invoked departed mothers. One, which is captioned "When women outlive their ovaries," depicts a sturdy white-haired woman who is apparently the proprietor of a country general store and gas station. Unlike the harpy, she is smiling. She doesn't need Premarin because she is already on it. "I saw what happened to my mother," she says. "It wasn't just how she looked. There was her back, stiff and bent . . . bladder trouble. I dreaded it."

McKenna's alluring fountain of youth had morphed into a house of horrors where women who "outlived their ovaries" were so useless they deserved to die. They would go bonkers without Premarin, dry up like prunes, pee in their diapers, and grow humpbacks while their bones crumbled into dust. The new slogan, "Keep Her on Premarin," was authoritarian, and women who refused to obey were described as "noncompliant." In her middle age, the sassy feminist author Germaine Greer was invited to give a keynote speech at a convention of gynecologists. She strode to the podium, placed her hands on her hips, and introduced herself: "Gentlemen, you see before you a noncompliant woman."

In the 1960s, the competition among popular-advice physicians heated up over who could insult mature women the most. In his 1969 best-seller, *Everything You Always Wanted to Know About Sex*, psychiatrist David Reuben appeared as insensitive as his predecessor by three years, Dr. Robert Wilson, author of *Feminine Forever*. It's true that in his book Wilson tossed out some nasty terms, such as *living decay*, but in person he seemed avuncular. He was quite eccentric and once confided to me, "There are some people who don't like me. They say I shouldn't do what I'm doing. They say that menopause is a natural process. We should grow old gracefully and enjoy it." He warmed to his topic. "They say we should do nothing to retard menopause. Just think of that. Isn't that dreadful? The estrogen regimen should start at age nine—nine to ninety. It's necessary to begin then and to check your estrogen level all through life, so that it never leaves you. Don't allow it to."

I asked Dr. Wilson to comment on the risks of endometrial cancer. "That's the worst lie in the world," he said, "the worst fallacy. I have over forty doctors working all over the world — Switzerland, Czechoslovakia, all over the world — and we haven't seen one case of cancer." However, when I criticized Wilson in print, he thanked me for the plug! "You spelled my name right," he said, and offered to "fix me up with estrogen free of charge."

As for Reuben, I've never understood why the hundreds of thousands of women who purchased *Everything You Always Wanted to Know About Sex* didn't march back to their bookstores and demand a refund when they read:

> As the estrogen is shut off a woman comes as close as she can to being a man. Increased facial hair, deepened voice, obesity, and the decline of breasts and female genitalia all contribute to a masculine appearance. Coarsened features, enlargement of the clitoris and gradual baldness increase the tragic picture. Not really a man but no longer a functional woman, these individuals live in the world of intersex.

Neither Wilson nor Reuben was particularly respected by their peers, but Wilson did enjoy the gratitude of many patients — and of Ayerst Laboratories as well — although in November 1966, he received a sharp slap on the wrist from the FDA, which pronounced him "unacceptable as an investigator for drugs in the menopause" because he was disseminating promotional material claiming hormones had been shown to be effective to "'prevent aging,' a condition for which they had never been proved to work." Not incidentally, his Robert Wilson Research Foundation was sponsored by three drug firms — Ayerst, of course, and also Searle and Upjohn.

Washington Post reporter Morton Mintz uncovered that in 1964 Wilson received $17,000 from the Searle Foundation, $8,700 from Ayerst Labs, and $5,600 from the Upjohn Company. Today that would total the equivalent of $176,485.43 in purchasing power. For Searle, the manufacturer of Enovid, the first oral contraceptive, Wilson was attempting to show that staying on the Pill could prevent menopause. For Upjohn he was testing the use in menopause of Provera, their popular progestin.

Searle and Upjohn eventually dumped Wilson, but Ayerst maintained its association. When Premarin or Wilson himself came under attack, he intimated to his worried followers that the drug might be banned or declared a controlled substance. Fran L., a sixty-five-year-old patient, testified at FDA hearings that any attempts to limit the use of estrogen would be irresponsible, like "taking insulin away from a diabetic."

Fran L. went on to explain that Wilson "saved her life" when he started her on Premarin at age fifty. She became an advocate, and told the FDA that her "extensive correspondence attests to the fact that Premarin has saved families and prevented suicides."

When her testimony was finished, Fran L. was asked if it was true that she was diagnosed with cancer. She acknowledged that she had "had three breast lumps removed" and no longer uses Premarin on a regular basis, but "goes back on it when she cannot cope physically with menopause symptoms." Years later, in 2002, Wilson's son, Ron, would announce that his mother, too, had had breast cancer.

But do bear in mind that during the years when Wilson flourished, most women were taking Premarin in dosages of 2.5 mg (purple tablets) or 1.25 mg (yellow). These were up to eight times the strength of the products favored in the twenty-first century, 0.625 mg tablets (reddish) and 0.3 mg (green). Even so, in an article entitled "Do Standard Doses of Frequently Prescribed Drugs Cause Preventable Adverse Effects in Women?"

appearing in the Spring 2002 issue of the *Journal of the American Medical Women's Association,* Dr. Jay S. Cohen scolded the company now called Wyeth: "The manufacturer does produce a 0.3 mg pill, but in its popular combination preparation (Prempro) the lowest available dose of conjugated estrogens remains 0.625 mg. Recent studies have shown that the amount of medroxyprogesterone (Provera) in this combination product is also higher than needed by many women."

In remembrance of my aunt Sally, I fell into an unkind pattern of outing women who exaggerated the benefits they reaped from estrogen treatments.

"At fifty," Dr. Wilson stated, "women on ERT [estrogen replacement therapy] still look attractive in sleeveless dresses or tennis shorts."

"How do you know," I asked him, "that it isn't from the tennis?"

In April 1976, this was the state of knowledge, as summarized by Dr. J. Richard Crout, director of the FDA Bureau of Drugs: "There is . . . testimonial evidence but there really are no controlled studies or any objective evidence to indicate that estrogens have any benefit in helping women look and feel young."

In 1977, I asked a different kind of expert, Mallen de Santis, the beauty and health editor of *Cosmopolitan,* if she agreed with Dr. Crout. She did, and she went further:

"Many actresses and society women who have face-lifts and plastic surgery are reluctant to admit it. When they appear looking somewhat rejuvenated they are much more apt to hint that they owe their suddenly younger faces to a drug, because this is somehow considered more respectable. Then, too, sometimes the manufacturer might reward them. The actresses are used to that way of life, making secret 'endorsements,' because they get compensation from the cigarette companies for smoking on the screen."

De Santis was in the business of interviewing professional beauties on their regimens. "They don't take estrogen seriously as a youth preservative. Some of them take it for hot flashes and other symptoms, but they have no illusion about its ability to improve their looks. These women can't afford to fool themselves because their livings depend on their looks."

One day I found myself on a lively TV program hosted by Barbara Walters called *Not for Women Only*. One of the other panelists was Dr. Mary Calderone, the photogenic daughter of photographer Edward Steichen and a well-known physician who had founded SEICUS (Sex Education and Information Council of the United States). When the subject of estrogen came up, Calderone declared that she took it, and people told her she looked good for her age. Correction: She didn't just "look good." She was a gorgeous white-haired grandmother. Just before the show, another panelist, sex therapist Dr. Helen Kaplan, whispered to me, "I'm trying to get the name of the surgeon who did Mary's face-lift; would you happen to know?"

Did you ever hear words coming out of your mouth that seem disconnected from your brain? I had one of those moments. When Calderone gave her plug for Premarin, I asked, "But didn't you also have a face-lift?"

She admitted it, but she was so humiliated that to this day I feel regretful. In retrospect, I often think I wouldn't have asked her that question, and yet sometimes when I consider how many millions of women still take this proven carcinogen for no good reason, I think I did the right thing. David Sackett, the great Canadian epidemiologist who was a major force in revealing that most tonsillectomies are unnecessary, spoke for me when he responded to the 2002 halting of the Prempro trial in an editorial he called "The Arrogance of Preventive Medicine," and he didn't mean your grandmother's caution to wear your galoshes in the rain or eat an apple a day.

> Preventive medicine displays all three elements of arrogance. First it is aggressively assertive, pursuing asymptomatic individuals and telling them what they must do to remain healthy. . . . Second, preventive medicine is presumptuous, confident that the interventions it espouses will, on average, do more good than harm to those who accept and adhere to them. Finally preventive medicine is overbearing, attacking those who question the value of its recommendations.

DR. ROBERT WILSON'S *FEMININE FOREVER*

"Thanks to my late father, a drug made from animal waste is the most widely prescribed drug in the world today."

— RON WILSON, *animal-rights activist*

Dr. Robert A. Wilson died in 1981, by his own hand. His wife, Thelma, died of breast cancer in 1988. Their younger son, Ron, of Cary, North Carolina, an animal-rights activist who is no fan of his father's book *Feminine Forever*, vouches that the catchy title was the youth-doctor's own creation, more or less. The son remembers when Robert and his collaborator exclaimed, "Eureka, we found a title." The lines that produced it appear on page 15 of the published book: A woman is not "complete" unless she takes hormone replacement pills. She will "be condemned to witness the death of her own womanhood." She cannot be "forever feminine" unless she takes hormone-replacement therapy. "Forever feminine" was inverted and, voilà, the campaign to "Keep her on Premarin" was launched.

McKenna's successors massaged *Feminine Forever* into a household word. The book had a short life span, and who knows how few read it now—there is little in it worth reading—but many still cling to the beautiful dream of staying young and sexy. The folks at what was then called Ayerst Laboratories, or American Home Products (Wyeth, you will remember, was a sister corporation owned by AHP), helped fund the writing of *Feminine Forever,* provided Wilson with editorial assistance, and even surreptitiously bought enough copies at retail to push it onto the bestseller lists. They kept the name of his book "in currency" long after the last copies disappeared from the remainder bins. A well-crafted excerpt in *Look* magazine was read by millions, and created quite a buzz.

But as for the book itself, it was hard, even then, to see how any woman could take it seriously. I'd hoped to give *Feminine Forever* a break because I'd reported only the negatives on estrogen—the uterine cancer from Premarin and the blood clots on the high-dose birth control pills. I was looking to balance my take on the situation with something positive . . . if only I could find it. On a blustery day in January 1966, I went to my little cubby at the *Ladies' Home Journal* to find myself the recipient of three copies of *Feminine Forever,* one from M. Evans Company, the publisher, one from the Robert A. Wilson Foundation, and one from the publicist at Ayerst. Here is an excerpt:

> It was quite late in the evening, toward the end of my consulting hours, when my receptionist told me there was a man in the waiting room who wished to see me. Male patients being a rarity

in a gynecologist's practice, I agreed to talk to him, even though he had come without an appointment.

A skinny man in his fifties with a sharp and sallow face slid rather furtively through the door. His manner was an unpleasant mixture of embarrassment and aggressiveness. For a while he just fidgeted, then, "Doc, they tell me you can fix women when they get old and crabby."

I sidestepped the implied question and let him tell more of his story:

"She's driving me nuts. She won't fix meals. She lets me get no sleep. She picks on me all the time. She makes up lies about me. She hits the bottle all day. And we used to be happily married. She's been to three doctors already," he continued. "They all tell her it's the change and nothing can be done about it. Now she tells me to get out and never come back. But I won't. It's my home. And if anyone's going she is."

He reached into his back pocket—in those days shoulder holsters were still unknown—and quietly laid a .32 automatic on the edge of my desk.

"If you don't cure her, I'll kill her."

I looked at him doubtfully. "You think that would be better for you?" I asked cautiously, my mind reeling with all I had heard about armed madmen in doctors' offices. But I was wrong. The man was completely rational.

"I got advanced T.B.," my visitor explained. "I was x-rayed again just last week. My doctor tells me that I have less than a year to live. I want to die in peace—and I can't if she's around."

> My client, I later discovered, was a prominent member of the
> Brooklyn underworld. . . . I accepted his wife as a patient. . . .
> Her disposition improved noticeably after three weeks, and soon
> she was very busy taking care of her sick husband.

This may sound like a script from a low-budget movie, but in fact it's an actual anecdote from one of the most influential so-called medical books of the past forty years.

Ron Wilson has compiled a list of twenty-one obnoxious statements from his father's book. Some examples: "The tragedy of menopause often destroys her character along with her health" (p. 20). "She becomes a 'dull-minded but sharp tongued caricature of her former self'"(p. 97). "When she realizes she is no longer a woman she may 'subside into a stupor of indifference'" (p. 44).

According to some calculations, Premarin sales tripled in the wake of *Feminine Forever*. Others say that sales merely doubled. In any event, they stayed at a record-breaking level until the mid-1970s, when they fell back temporarily. You might wonder, how could Ayerst Labs have obtained so much mileage from such a shallow book? Not a mystery once the book was out of sight and they were left with just the tantalizing title. They also had the right woman at the right time on their promotion team: Sondra Gorney, who, for her efforts, won the coveted Matrix Award in 1973 as *the* outstanding New York woman in the field of public relations. Gorney, who had been a dancer in her youth, made a successful comeback as an actress after her retirement from Ayerst, appearing in numerous off-Broadway original plays, repertory theater, and commercials and on television. She is widely admired as a grande dame, an accomplished woman of a certain age who looks at least twenty years younger and has more energy than her granddaughters.

You may be wondering, "Does Sondra Gorney take Premarin?" The answer is "Yes, but . . . She goes to a health club three times a week, spends a half hour on the bike, twenty minutes on a treadmill, ten or fifteen minutes on a rowing machine, then takes an hour calisthenics class, which includes light aerobics, stretching, and weight lifting. She also walks a lot." Gorney had not been on Premarin continuously. She went off for a time and then went back on.

Remember when a popular ad for hair dye was "Does she or doesn't she? Only her hair dresser knows for sure"? Ho-hum. No one cares anymore. Now we take it for granted that most women do. The new burning question, especially when we meet a spectacular older woman, is "Does she or doesn't she . . . take Premarin?" Sondra Gorney does now, and certainly she knows a great deal about the product, but as I once asked Dr. Wilson, "Could it be the tennis?"

How did Sondra Gorney (still fabulous at eighty-five, still keeping herself on Premarin) legitimize and iconize the philosophy of *Feminine Forever* for a decade after its publication? Her job title at the time was executive director of the Information Center on the Mature Woman, a "service for media" provided by Ayerst Labs and located in New York City. Those were the days that the PMA (Pharmaceutical Manufacturers Association, now widely nicknamed Big Pharma) subscribed to a code of ethics maintaining that prescription drugs would not be advertised directly to the public. Never mind; for the price of Gorney's salary, a fraction of what Ayerst would have spent to *buy* the space, magazine and newspaper editors frequently published features supplied by Gorney. Her style was breezy and readable but authoritative, and she always dealt with up-to-date menopause questions and controversies. Gorney's free newsletters and "background papers" were attributed, if at all, to the Information Center on the Mature Woman, even though, to Gorney's credit, her mailings to the media did acknowledge the Ayerst support. Gorney's information center closed in 1976, but the beat goes on.

THE JIG IS UP

On November 20, 2002, reporter Sharyl Attkisson "outed" two of most widely quoted menopause experts, Drs. Lila Nachtigall and Wulf Utian, on the *CBS Evening News*, making them publicly acknowledge their receipt of financial support from the makers of Premarin and other hormones. Just four weeks earlier, at a scientific workshop on menopausal hormone therapy at the NIH, Drs. Nachtigall and Utian both signed a "Disclosure Statement" required of all speakers, asking them to state whether or not they had any financial ties to drug companies. Eleven of the forty-nine presenters at the workshop acknowledged such connections, but neither Dr. Nachtigall nor Dr. Utian was among them. Both denied *any* conflict of interest, yet here is what Attkisson uncovered: "The selling of HRT was a coup . . . but a lot of the claims weren't backed by serious science . . . women never knew the same doctors promoting the wonders of HRT often had a vested interest in the drug's success. Much of the information that got into print was bolstered by quotes from respected experts such as Dr. Lila Nachtigall . . . Readers *weren't* told that Nachtigall is also a paid speaker for at least eleven drug companies including Wyeth — the biggest maker of HRT drugs. But Nachtigall says, 'I have ties to no one.' Dr. Wulf Utian, another widely quoted specialist who is Director of the North American Menopause Society, has, as it turns out, gotten large grants and support from Wyeth. Though he says he's staunchly unbiased, he agrees that 'when you see a magazine article and see a quotation from an expert, I think it's almost impossible to know whether there's a conflict-of-interest or not.' "

So, now he tells us!

CHAPTER 4

A DARING PROGRAM TO KEEP
WOMEN YOUNG

You are among the first people to have access to these new things.

— DR. ROBERT B. GREENBLATT to his patients

Flashback now to 1938, which proved to be a bountiful year in the estrogen business. It was the year when Charlie Dodds published his formula for stilbestrol in *Nature* magazine, when Adolph Butenandt's colleagues completed the paperwork on the ethinyl estradiol patents, when Bill McKenna or an associate at Ayerst came up with Premarin's unforgettable name. And it was the year that the Greatest Experiment had officially commenced, launched by the publication of two major papers on hot flashes. The first, in *JAMA*, was titled "The Menopausal Syndrome: One Thousand Consecutive Patients Treated with Estrogen." The second, in *Endocrinology*, was called "The Menopause: A Consideration of the Symptoms, Etiology, and Treatment by Means of Estrogens." Both studies confirmed the benefits of estrogen in curbing hot flashes, and both warned that long-term use of these drugs might be carcinogenic. Neither paper suggested in any way that estrogen could delay aging.

The idea of a fountain of youth would be introduced by two young doctors: The first was Robert Benjamin Greenblatt, a firm believer in wonder drugs derived from his own heralded research on antibiotics, and the second was Fuller Albright, a Harvard genius in declining health who maintained, "Any theory is better than no theory at all." Neither were household names, but by the power of their prestige and impressive research, as well as the students they trained to carry on their work, they lent academic credibility to the dream that artificial hormones could keep women young.

Dr. Robert Benjamin Greenblatt graduated first in his class at McGill University Medical School in 1932. Like other students, he had a burning interest in the new science of hormones and endocrinology, inspired largely by James Bertram Collip of the biochemistry department, who, having discovered insulin, was now working on early versions of the estrogen product that would become Premarin. Greenblatt expected to stay at McGill for training, but instead he and his bride, the former Gwendolyn Lande, immigrated to the United States, where he specialized in gynecology. In 1935, he applied for a faculty job at the Medical College of Georgia and was hired by its president, Lombard Kelly, who had declared, "There's going to be something to endocrinology," words that were music to Greenblatt's eager ears.

Soon after he arrived in Augusta, Greenblatt was called upon to investigate granuloma inguinale, a venereal disease endemic in the South. In the process of his research he discovered that mycins could cure the disease, and as a result, it almost disappeared, a major public-health conquest for him and for the region. In wartime 1942, Greenblatt joined the Navy and was sent to Savannah to save the region from yet another venereal-disease epidemic—this one rampant among sailors and their families. Next, he was assigned to Hot Springs, Arkansas, to work on a crash government program similar to the Manhattan Project but designed to develop penicillin. Finally, Greenblatt, by now a commander, joined the Pacific fleet, where, after three ships were torpedoed out from under him, he participated in the invasion of Okinawa, ran a hospital on the beach, and was one of the first scientists to investigate the effects of the atom bomb at Nagasaki.

But Greenblatt never stopped obsessing over hormones or dreaming of becoming head of the first endocrinology department at an American medical school, a position Kelly had offered to consider him for after the war. Torpedoes might besiege him, atomic bombs might be dropped, but the unsinkable gynecologist from Augusta would keep up his writing schedule. In 1943, Greenblatt published two electrifying articles, one in *JAMA* and the other in the *Journal of Clinical Endocrinology*, on the benefits of testosterone pellets he had implanted in fifty-five female patients. The latter article, called "Hormone Factors in Libido," gives us a snapshot of the man and his mind:

> Seventy-five to 200 mg of testosterone has frequently proved aphrodisiacal. Many married women volunteered the information that the loss of sexual desire led to marital discord. Following pellet implantation there was a return of coital pleasure, which often terminated in orgasm. A reawakened interest on the part of the husband usually followed, and husband and wife once more fell in love.

Female orgasms. Falling in love. You don't often see discussions like this in medical journals, not even now, and surely not back in that pre–Alfred Kinsey era. Greenblatt's was truly a breakthrough report. He signed off with four conclusions that still hold up today;

> 1.   *From the inconsistent evidence now available a final over-all appraisal of the precise significance of hormonal factors in libido cannot be offered.*
>
> 2.   *Human behavior involves all sorts of mental processes not subject to experimental control. In women with normal libido, sexual gratification may depend mostly on the proper "amatory prelude" or on the proper mechanics of coitus.*
>
> 3.   *Sufficient evidence has accumulated to show that the administration to women of estrogenic and particularly andro-genic substances in sufficient dosage may increase or awaken libido. . . .*
>
> 4.   *Altogether, it appears then, that sexual libido is a phenome-non depending in part but not entirely upon well defined chemi-cal substances.*

Lombard Kelly kept his promise, and in 1946, at age forty, Greenblatt saw his dreamed-of life, based on hard work and great discoveries, open before him: He was appointed chief of endocrinology at the Medical College of Georgia. Here was a man who understood his limitations, regretting that he had no doctorate in biochemistry to add to his M.D., but as chairman of his own endocrinology department, Greenblatt was free now to recruit gifted associates. One in particular, Virendra B. Mahesh from India, with double Ph.D. degrees in chemistry and biological sciences, would become his frequent research partner, the Hammerstein to his Rodgers, and—being twenty-five years younger—would become departmental chair when Greenblatt stepped down in 1972.

Greenblatt also enlisted help from his relatives. Edward, his middle child, now a lawyer in Atlanta, recalls that between the ages of ten and twelve, he earned his pocket money by performing his father's pregnancy tests. "We had these little mice. We injected them with a patient's urine. We sacrificed the mice and looked at the ovaries. If they were inflamed the patient was pregnant." Greenblatt's wife, Gwendolyn, also had an important role to play. When her husband was out of town, which was often, she prescribed for his patients. They would call her and she would call the pharmacist, who had been instructed by Greenblatt to fill his wife's orders.

The first I heard of Dr. Robert B. Greenblatt was at a New York party in 1963, when I was introduced to a woman and her daughter from the royal family of Iran. They were on their way to Augusta to consult the great physician—the mother for her "change of life," the daughter for help in getting pregnant. For thirty-five years, after his mornings of teaching and before his evenings of making hospital rounds and then retiring to his study to write for hours, Greenblatt treated twenty to thirty patients a day, five days a week, in his private practice.

The airlines that flew into Augusta and the city's hotels owed the doctor an enormous debt of gratitude for all the business he generated. He was a highly successful fertility specialist, training scores of men and women who are still eminent today. Some, such as Paul McDonough, president of the American Fertility Society and editor of its journal, are quietly powerful. Others, unfortunately, overreached. Ricardo Asch, for one, was dismissed from his professorship at the University of California for misappropriating human eggs, making embryos, and then transferring them to other patients.

Greenblatt's costly made-to-order pellet implants, featuring a variety of hormone products in a range of dosages designed to remain active for three to six months or more, were much appreciated by his midlife patients. But he mocked himself when these women grew too fulsome or treated him like a god. "Touch my robe," he would quip, and "you'll be cured." Virendra Mahesh recalls Greenblatt as "kind, helpful, and imposing." I think it was his private practice that helped to keep him pure and relatively independent of drug-company influence. He did experiment with patients in a way that might be frowned on today, but his was a different era, characterized by more faith and trust in medical progress, and Greenblatt, so familiar with the miracle that insulin really was, so successful in his own research on antibiotic wonder drugs, could not but believe that the right combination of hormones, as he and his gifted staff might show the world one day, could preserve a woman's youthfulness and sexuality and prolong her life.

Unlike other medications with a narrower range of impact, hormones have an effect on every cell and every organ in the body. Greenblatt never deceived his patients that what he was giving them experimentally was tried and true. On the contrary, he made a virtue of their novelty. His patients were impressed and even thrilled when he informed them that they were "among the first people to have access to these new things."

In high school Latin classes, I learned that "all Gaul is divided into three parts." Ten years later, I heard Greenblatt lecture that "all menopause is divided into three kinds of miseries." The first and most common were hot flashes, sweats, palpitations, spasms, and something called globus hystericus, "a subjective sensation of a lump in the throat, a condition frequently seen in hysteria." The second miseries were mood disturbances—apprehension, depression, insomnia, and nervousness—

along with headaches and frigidity. The third were metabolic disorders, particularly osteoporosis and muscle pain. Greenblatt was careful to point out that bone loss should "not be regarded solely as an aging process. It occurs in much younger women after extirpation [removal] of the ovaries also known as oophorectomy or ovariectomy, the equivalent of castration in the male." He credited Fuller Albright for making this discovery.

HOW TO EXTIRPATE AND IMPLANT

Shortly before I met Dr. Greenblatt, I heard him give one of his famous lectures on the blissful benefits of testosterone pellets, a theory he'd developed twenty years earlier and of which he was still an advocate. His favorite prescription for women who'd had their ovaries "extirpated" was a combination of two 2.5 mg pellets of estradiol and one 75 mg pellet of testosterone, to be renewed twice a year. Pellets could be implanted by incision or with a special instrument called a Kearns pellet injector. The sites for implantation were armpits, the region of the shoulder blades, sometimes the abdomen, or internally during surgery at the time the ovaries were "extirpated." It's hard for me to restrain myself from writing "at the time of castration." People don't like to hear the word, but it's an accurate description of the procedure. When women know that fact, fewer agree to it.

In his lectures, Greenblatt always acknowledged the common side effects of hormone therapy: uterine bleeding, pelvic congestion, edema, weight gain, sore breasts. Other doctors would cite further side effects observed from their practices: nausea, spider veins, spotted skin. Without seeming arrogant, Greenblatt would divulge how he adjusted hormone products and dosages to the individual, or how, when needed, he might add further medications to reduce unpleasant side effects. He was one for running lots of additional tests. He tinkered. He tweaked. I fully believe that, given time, he succeeded in making most of his patients comfortable, even "in the pink." (An interesting fact I learned from observing Greenblatt is that rich women had more fun at menopause. They could fly to Augusta twice a year for their implantations, combining the trip with a golf holiday.)

Greenblatt wrote a popular manual called *Office Endocrinology.* He could share his knowledge, but not necessarily his skills, and certainly not his intuition. He was most likely the greatest "manager" of long-term hormone therapy who ever lived.

Is Menopause a Transition or a Sentence for Life?

On the one hand, Greenblatt laid down the basis for doctors to call menopause a deficiency disease. Of course, he himself put it more guardedly: "Although the menopause is a physiologic process and represents a period of adjustment to a new *milieu interieur*, it is a hormonal-deficiency state. . . . Our viewpoint . . . is that endocrine deficiency syndromes require endocrine replacement, and the menopause is no exception." At the same time, he didn't insist, certainly not to me, that every woman needed HRT: "There are many women who, although their menses cease, continue to have enough estrogen produced within the body to maintain a normal metabolic and nervous system balance. They do not have hot flashes. No evidence of estrogen lack is seen on vaginal cytology. In our view these women do not need to be treated." But at other times, Greenblatt sounded as if he expected all women to need hormones sooner or later. For example, "The difficulties of the menopause continue from mild to severe form until the end of life. It is unrealistic to withhold measures that may make the transition smoother or prevent disabling pathologic processes."

Years after Greenblatt's death, I asked Virendra Mahesh which way the wind really blew for his colleague. He replied, "Bob advocated that not everyone should be treated, but he really believed that everyone should." I wasn't surprised. I appreciate that Greenblatt took care not to be too pushy.

Greenblatt was not a tyrant, but I did have a serious bone to pick with him. Not only did he practice denial on the cancer risks, he sometimes went so far as to claim that estrogens are "capable of inducing regressions in breast cancer, particularly in postmenopausal women." For some years, he went back and forth on the use of progestins to prevent endometrial cancer, but in a 1979 article, published in the *Journal of the American Geriatrics Society*, he acknowledged that this cancer could be avoided "if regular cyclic courses of an oral progestin are added to the regimen."

By the time of his death in 1987 from lung cancer (yes, he had smoked until the Surgeon General's report in 1964), Greenblatt had published six hundred articles, written or edited twenty-five books and ninety-five chapters in the medical literature, and contributed eighteen essays on endocrinology to the *Encyclopaedia Britannica*. He also wrote a popular book called *Search the Scriptures: A Physician Examines Medicine in the Bible*, published in 1963 and reprinted twenty-seven times.

What was *Search the Scriptures* about? Endocrine problems, of course, and how they altered the course of history. Take Esau, for example, who was forced to sell his birthright for a mess of pottage. Well, he had to, Greenblatt concluded. Poor Esau was so severely hypoglycemic that he could have died without that snack.

Greenblatt held a long-term stake in the future of hormone treatments, in the inbred fashion that only the powerful head of a university department or a very great teacher can do. He disliked "surgical solutions" if they could be avoided, a reason he gave for his proactive notions on using strong medicine instead. One time in the 1970s, when my friend Rose Kushner mounted a campaign against radical mastectomies, an operation named after the surgeon William Halsted, I asked Greenblatt if he agreed that this kind of mutilating surgery went too far. He said Kushner might be right in agitating for trials against less debilitating procedures. But why, I asked, are the "big" surgeons trying to sabotage the clinical trials that Kushner pushed for? Why wouldn't they want to compare the effectiveness of lumpectomies against radical mastectomies?

His answer stunned me. It was something I should have known but never thought of. It explains why Greenblatt has left permanent fingerprints and remains a progenitor of the theory of youth through long-term hormone treatments. He explained that Halsted "was the founder of the first department of surgery at an American medical school, Johns Hopkins, in the 1890s. He trained the next generation of academic surgeons. His residents fanned out to other great institutions, and they in turn trained the generation that followed."

I was getting it. "Do you mean that . . . "

"Yes, Ms. Seaman, I mean that your 'big' surgeons of today were trained by the men who were trained by Halsted. It's like patricide for them to support Ms. Kushner and go against radical mastectomy." William Halsted died in 1922, but fifty years later, his theory still ruled breast surgery.

Now I understood what drove Greenblatt to work constantly—all that teaching and administrative detail on top of his huge practice, his research, and the demanding writing schedule he set for himself every night. To a man as idea-driven as he, students represented his immortality. They would see that his work lived on. And they have seen to it. That is, until 2002, when the evidence seemed to turn against standard long-term therapy.

What would he say today with all of the evidence against hormone therapy? I can't see him letting his ego stand in the way of accepting reality. He was a good enough scientist that I would like to think that he would dig right in to do the research we need now, identifying those women who really do benefit from hormone treatments.

With Mahesh, his major collaborator, Greenblatt laid the groundwork for understanding hirsutism and polycystic ovaries, pioneered the use of Clomid to treat infertility, showed how progesterone receptors function in the ovary, discovered and reported that normal ovaries secrete some androgens and that hormones continue to be manufactured in the postmenopausal ovary. His work on STDs was of the highest order, and one wishes he were here today to wrestle with the new ones. We might seek clues from his classic 1940s monographs for the U.S. Public Health Service. Well before Greenblatt snatched Mahesh from Yale in 1959—in preparation for some of his greatest work—he had compiled a formidable record. For example, in 1946 he developed the "delay of menses" test, to interpret the strength and action of hormone products. He showed that if you give estrogen, the endometrium starts to grow, while progesterone makes it ready for implantation and prevents withdrawal bleeding. Greenblatt used this knowledge to develop new ways for treating a wide variety of "woman troubles," including painful menstruation and irregularities. In 1954 he showed that a combination of hormones, equivalent to those that would soon be incorporated into birth control pills, could stop ovulation, thus easing the pain of certain menstrual disorders.

Greenblatt learned his science during the decades between the great wars, when it seemed that every new discovery, from insulin to penicillin, really was a wonder drug, and like others of his generation, he may have harbored too much faith in where it all might lead. But just as Halsted will always be remembered as one of our greatest surgeons, Greenblatt and his partner, Dr. Mahesh, will be remembered for breakthroughs in the areas of antibiotics, menstruation, ovaries, and infertility.

CHAPTER 5

CRAZY PEOPLE IN AMERICA

Any theory is better than no theory at all.

— DR. FULLER ALBRIGHT to his students

There was hardly a day in 1938 when Charlie Dodds didn't get news of someone hatching plans to experiment with his brand-new estrogen. Puzzling him most were "some crazy people in America" who, from Boston to Texas, seemed to be embracing diethylstilbestrol, or DES, as the new frontier. Charlie Dodds, a physician as well as a biochemist, kept his functions impeccably separate. You do your experiments in your laboratory, never on your patients. But there was this Texas fellow, Karl John Karnaky, a wealthy man who ran his own clinic, with no trustees or review board to question his methods of injecting stilbestrol directly into the wombs of pregnant women to prevent miscarriages. Dodds was so distressed and even sickened by Karnaky's methods that he felt duty-bound to run his own trials on pregnant rabbits and rats. Once again he rushed the results into print, this time in the *British Medical Journal* on September 10, 1938, reporting that the early administration of stilbestrol would prevent implantation of a fertilized egg in the uterus, or if the pregnancy was already established, the hormone would end it. To make sure that no one misunderstood, he stated the obvious: "It is extremely probable that the factors governing the implantation of the fertilized egg are fundamentally similar in women and lower animals."

Apparently, none of this stopped Karnaky, but thirty years later Dodds's words did catch the eye of Dr. Louise Kuchera of the University of Michigan Health Services, who promoted DES as a "morning-after" contraceptive and claimed that, in a sample of 1,000 women, no pregnancies resulted—research that Belita Cowan, a college health instructor and cofounder of the National Women's Health Network, discovered was flawed. On February 27, 1975, Edward Kennedy invited Cowan to testify at his Senate hearing on her survey of over 200 patients. She said, "The most interesting finding of the study is that 24 percent of the women stated that they did not take all ten pills in the series. As one woman put it, 'I got so sick from the first pill that I never took the rest. I couldn't stand to be that ill.'"

Charlie Dodds had died by this point. Perhaps it was just as well, because it seemed the whenever he tried to put his genie back in the bottle, things only got worse.

Compared to the likes of Karnaky, Fuller Albright was held in relatively high regard by Dodds. After all, Albright was a creative, out-of-the-box thinker who, like Dodds himself, was curious to see exactly what stilbestrol might do for females who lacked ovaries. Albright got hooked on two apparently unrelated findings. The first was that in preparation for egg laying, pigeons and other fowl show an increase in osteoblastic activity (i.e., bone formation). In other words, for the time being, their bones get stronger and less breakable. His other discovery was that women whose ovaries are surgically removed in their twenties or early thirties often lose bone mass so fast they may develop osteoporosis before the age of forty. Putting these findings together, Albright proposed that estrogen might stimulate bone formation, and he soon launched the world's first experiment on the role of estrogen in osteoporosis. With his colleagues Patricia Smith and Anna Richardson, he published his review of forty-two cases of osteoporosis in the *JAMA* in 1941. We don't know if the decision to tread lightly was made by the authors or the editors at the journal, but someone decided not to use the word *estrogen* in the title, instead calling the piece "Postmenopausal Osteoporosis: Its Clinical Features." Perhaps it was feared that the suggestion of long-term treatments could set off alarm bells among the coterie of doctors busy documenting estrogen's carcinogenic effects. But the understanding was that the report was venturing into uncharted waters, recommending not only a long-term therapy but also a youth pill! "There is considerable evidence," it stated with an uncharacteristic lack of documentation, "that patients with postmenopausal osteoporosis have a tendency to atrophy of other tissues, notably the skin."

JAMA readers may have been intrigued by Albright's theory, but they were not convinced. It was a long and circuitous route from pigeon hens to women with fractures of the hip or spine. As distinguished as Albright was destined to become, his theories on estrogen and bone formation fanned few fires in 1941. Acclaim would have to wait five years, until Navy Commander Robert Greenblatt returned from Japan, his A-bomb investigations behind him, ready for happier projects, such as testing Albright's long-term protocols on his own patients, as well as popularizing them to adventurous gynecologists. Greenblatt's son, Edward, counting the references in his father's influential book *Office Endocrinology*, discovered that he cited Albright more than any other source.

Nonetheless, for forty years the FDA verdict on estrogen vis-à-vis osteoporosis was "possibly effective," meaning the agency was open-minded but less than convinced. It would not be until a 1984 landmark Consensus Conference that the NIH and FDA came to view estrogen as "probably effective," which was still short of saying, "We know for sure that it works." Here is a middle-of-the-road assessment dated 1973. It's from *Medical Letter*, the *Consumer Reports* of prescription drugs:

> Routine use of estrogens in menopausal patients for prevention or treatment of osteoporosis continues to be recommended by some experienced clinicians, but in the opinion of a majority of *Medical Letter* consultants there is no convincing evidence that estrogen administration reduces the loss of bone mass in aging women. Calcium balance often becomes positive early in the course of estrogen administration in osteoporotic patients, but long-term treatment is accompanied by a less positive or a return to a negative calcium balance, and it is possible that long-term estrogen treatment may ultimately result in decreased bone formation.

Estrogen to treat osteoporosis would not be credited as one of Fuller Albright's more successful discoveries until it was far too late for him to know about it. In the year 2000, the hundredth anniversary of his birth, he would be commemorated at scientific meetings all over the world as *the* father of metabolic bone research. Dr. Alois Alzheimer had only one disease named for him, and Dr. Henry Heimlich one maneuver, but Fuller Albright was so prolific that a dozen diseases or procedures bore his name, including Albright's syndrome and Albright's test. But his estrogen/osteoporosis thesis more or less languished until the early 1980s, although Robert Greenblatt remained a loyal advocate, keeping the ball in play with enthusiastic references to Albright's theory in his own articles and books.

At last, in 1982, a small but beautifully designed study by a San Francisco radiologist, Harry Genant, changed all that—more than either Albright or Genant might have wished. Genant's classic paper, published in the *Annals of Internal Medicine*, had a name that doesn't roll off the tongue: "Quantitative Computed Tomography of Vertebral Spongiosa: A Sensitive Method for Detecting Early Bone Loss after Oophorectomy." Don't worry, the research is easier to understand than the title. Genant recruited thirty-seven volunteers who were all still menstruating at the time they had their ovaries removed, plunging them into a surgical menopause. An expert on bone densitometry, Genant had access to new and top-notch highly sensitive measuring equipment and was able to meticulously trace their retention of bone mass. In a random, double-blind study, nine patients received placebo; six received a 0.625 mg dose of estrogen (the same amount as in the Prempro pills in the halted arm of the WHI study). The remaining volunteers received lower doses of Premarin. Dr. Genant took measurements over a twenty-four-month span. His finding: The women on 0.625 mg of Premarin retained their bone mass far better than those on lower doses or placebo. This was excellent news for women who'd had oophorectomies. If they experienced rapid bone loss, as many would, they could be identified early on and protected with an adequate dose of estrogen.

But, alas, as often happened in the Greatest Experiment, when a study was actually performed—however watertight it may have been—its results were extended and ballyhooed beyond what was justified. Something got lost in translation—the truth. Word went out that rapid bone loss at menopause could be held at bay with 0.625 mg of Premarin, but the term *oophorectomy* was not always included. Genant confirmed Albright's thesis—as Dodds had long expected—in patients without ovaries, *but not necessarily in patients undergoing natural menopause*, contrary to what most of us were led to believe. Dropping this distinction was a Machiavellian marketing trick. Genant's 1982 report states: "Albright in 1940 first described the importance of loss of ovarian function in the evolution of postmenopausal osteoporosis . . . Our data show that, in women studied early after oophorectomy . . . 0.6 mg is effective in almost all women." In September 2002, in response to my queries, Dr. Genant wrote to me: "I thought it was generally clear what the target population was. Surgical menopause brings about more abrupt and greater bone loss."

Even today, how many women are told the unvarnished truth before they agree to ovarian surgery? The radical operation, of which 300,000 per year are performed in the United States, is a great boost to hormone sales. Fifty percent of the women who have surgical menopause wind up staying on estrogen for the rest of their lives, while only some 10 percent of those who've gone through natural menopause do so. After Genant's initial research made its splash, I awaited the follow-up. His findings could have been publicized to deter women from ovarian castration unless there was good reason, and also to better target the patients most likely to benefit from estrogen. But that, I knew, was not how the system worked. In April 1984, the National Institutes of Health convened a Consensus Development Conference on Osteoporosis. It was chaired by Dr. William Peck, professor (and later dean) at the Washington University School of Medicine in St. Louis, who would become a paid adviser to a manufacturer of bone-densitometry equipment. The report from Dr. Peck's conference urged that low-dosage measuring devices, less expensive than Dr. Genant's, be developed and made readily available. A rush to get FDA approval followed, as did a fiasco in which, according to Dr. Suzanne Parisian, formerly of the agency's Bureau of Medical Devices, questionable equipment was "grandfathered" in (without testing), based on similarities to earlier equipment that was never proved reliable in the first place, so that women were subjected to aggressive marketing and exposure to a decade of unreliable and sometimes dangerous bone-measurement devices. It's clear that Albright would have been thrilled at Genant's work but appalled at some of what came after.

Born in Buffalo to wealthy parents, Fuller Albright had a stunning if tragic life, becoming a victim of Parkinson's disease when he was but thirty-six years old. He graduated from Harvard Medical School in 1924, specialized in internal medicine at Johns Hopkins, and then sailed off to Europe to sharpen his skills. He went to Germany, the place to go for avant-garde science in the years between the two great wars. When he returned to Harvard in 1930, Albright founded a biological laboratory as well as an endocrinology clinic at Metabolic Ward 4 of Massachusetts General Hospital. He added a clinic for ovarian function and another for kidney stones, which he nicknamed "the quarry."

In 1946, at their twenty-fifth reunion, Fuller Albright wrote to his Harvard College classmates: "Over the last ten years I have had the interesting experience of observing the course of Parkinson's syndrome on myself. This condition in fact does not belong to my special medical interests or else I am certain I would have solved it long ago."

When Albright began his stilbestrol experiments in 1938, he was already two years into his Parkinson's diagnosis. At first, he "kept an extraordinary mental clearness while his motor capacity deteriorated." With the help of his wife, Claire, his many disciples, and his medical students, who vied for the honor of providing him monthly wheelchair duty, he continued to work at almost his normal pace—until the early 1950s.

In June 1956, he decided to undergo an experimental brain operation called chemopallidectomy—a daring attempt at a better life. The intervention on the right side freed him from tremor, enabling him to stand and walk a bit and to use his hand. A second operation was followed by a massive intracranial hemorrhage, causing him to never speak again. He slipped into unconsciousness and remained in a room at Massachusetts General Hospital for thirteen years until his death.

Dodds respected Albright but worried when his American counterpart crossed the line, treating some women who'd had natural menopauses along with those who'd had surgical removal of their ovaries, a faux pas that Albright's disciple, Harry Genant, would not make. Also, said Dodds, Albright didn't go far enough, in that he neglected to study the seesaw phenomenon—namely, that women and other mammals get more breast cancer when their bone mass is good, and less if their bones are thinning. Estrogen stimulates growth. Perhaps it stimulates bone cells and cancer cells simultaneously. Some sort of inverse relation exists— that is, according to Dodds, you're more likely to get female cancers if your bones are hearty, less likely if they are delicate. But being that deaths from cancer start to occur far earlier in life than deaths from hip fracture, it seems presumptuous, Dodds believed, to give estrogen to prevent osteoporosis until you have figured out the relationship between the two.

"I feel I'm part of history."

— *PEGGY MURPHY, volunteer in the Women's Health Initiative*
Clinical Trial

In the summer of 2002, shortly after the Prempro arm of the NIH study called the Women's Health Initiative was halted, Dr. Sylvia W. Smoller, head of a branch of the study at the Albert Einstein College of Medicine in New York, invited me to sit in at a meeting she was holding for her newly "unblinded" volunteers. These women had been receiving either Prempro or a placebo for 5.2 years, expecting to continue for three more. All of the Prempro pills were of the same dosage, containing 0.625 mg of Premarin and 2.5 mg of Provera. However, NIH safety monitors discovered that the volunteers on Prempro, as compared to placebo, had more incidences of breast cancer, heart disease, stroke, and blood clots in their lungs and veins. As the risks outweighed the benefits, the researchers were required to stop the trial. JAMA posted the information on the Web on July 9 and published it July 17. Some prescribing doctors were outraged and skeptical, wondering whether, before the results were posted, someone should have tested if lower doses or other formulations might have proved felicitous. In a time-honored shoot-the-messenger tradition, Dr. Catherine DeAngelis, editor of JAMA, came under attack. "I'm getting letters saying, 'How dare you publish this without also publishing a rebuttal?' What rebuttal?" When HRT patients heard about the risks, and they did in front-page stories that dominated the health news for weeks, many felt betrayed by their doctors: "What should I do? I've been on hormone-replacement therapy for ten years and it sounds like I'm at risk of dying every minute I'm on it!" is how a reader of the *Harvard Women's Health Watch* put it.

However, at Dr. Smoller's meeting, most of her volunteers seemed the opposite of angry. They, too, were puzzled, asking technical questions, but they were also proud and in a way even spiritually lifted, as people are apt to be in the aftermath of a powerful good deed. They'd signed on, hoping to make a contribution to science, and they had! The size of the study and its truly unexpected ending gave exceptional importance to the discoveries. The women in the trial risked their own health to make these discoveries possible. As Dr. David Sackett put it in his editorial for the *Canadian Medical Association Journal*, "First place among the heroes is shared by each of the 16,608 women who agreed to collab-

One way of calculating *absolute* risks:

> Among 10,000 taking Prempro for one year, there will be 7
> more coronary heart disease events, 8 more invasive breast can-
> cers, 8 more strokes, and 8 more blood clots in the lung, but 6
> fewer colorectal cancers and 5 fewer hip fractures.

Great research often dispels myth. Benefits to the heart turned out to be a fairy tale, and I don't know that there was ever any major scientist at, say, the Albright level who showed up to vigorously support the claims for cardio fitness. But Albright's fracture-prevention theory, amazingly, still lives, even though competing products such as Fosamax and Actonel (bisphosphonates) have come along, and so has Evista (a selective estrogen receptor modulator, or SERM), leading Dr. Ethel Siris, director of the Osteoporosis Center at New York's Columbia Presbyterian, to declare: "In the twentieth century people had only two choices: They could take estrogen or they could not take estrogen. Now we have more choices for effective treatment."

People who run clinics are always on the lookout for new treatments. But in a more surprising move, announced September 4, 2002, Wyeth itself changed the prescribing recommendations for the Premarin family of products, preempting the FDA and moving to a more cautionary stance than the regulators were apt to require. Never in the entire history of Premarin has this reporter ever seen or heard of this drug company giving in on a new regulation *before* the FDA ordered it. I was stunned to read that the new labels on Premarin and its derivatives state: "When used solely for the prevention of postmenopausal osteoporosis, alternative treatments should be carefully considered." It's like

Hertz telling its customers, "Forget about us; you should consider Avis." It seems like a touching postscript to Fuller Albright's brilliant but tragic life that, just when his theory on estrogen and osteoporosis prevention was proven to full scientific satisfaction, the world had moved on to different and newer products.

CHAPTER 6

CENSORSHIP, CLASS-ACTION LAWSUITS, AND DANGEROUS OFF-LABEL PRESCRIPTION DRUGS

The public must realize that of what students learn in four years of medical school, only a third will still hold true; in ten years, one third will be completely disproven and one third will be controversial or problematic. Most of the public is being taken care of by physicians who are ten to thirty years out of medical school. Who is responsible for their re-education? All physicians must earn fifty hour credits of CME [continuing medical education] every year to renew their licenses. But nobody cares about the sponsorship of those courses.

—DR. LILA WALLIS

If there is a trusted and universally respected first lady of hormone research, it is likely Dr. Elizabeth Barrett-Connor, professor of family and preventive medicine at the University of California in San Diego. She is founder and director of the Rancho Bernardo Heart and Chronic Disease

WITHDRAWN

Study, now in its twenty-fifth year. She served as a principal investigator of the PEPI study (Postmenopausal Estrogen/Progestin Interventions) and the HERS study (Heart and Estrogen-Progestin Replacement Study), both forerunners of the Women's Health Initiative, for which she serves as a consultant. She was one of the first to discover that estrogen might prevent heart disease and also among the first to suggest that estrogen users, after all, might just be taking better care of themselves, as now seems to be the suspicion. By the 1990s, Wyeth had mastered advanced strategies and skills at using the power of its checkbook not only to advance its supporters but to silence its critics. It held great influence in the field of CME, where its enthusiasts, including Dr. Rogerio Lobo of Columbia University and Dr. Charles Hammond of Duke University, wrote and updated widely cir-culated CME courses on menopause and hormone topics. Five years ago, I was invited to attend a Barrett-Connor presentation at a meeting of the American Medical Women's Association. The doctor was to participate in a CME panel on menopause. I hadn't heard her speak in years and was look-ing forward to her arguments, as she was always at the forefront of estrogen research. To my disappointment, I learned that she would not appear after all. The reason: Wyeth-Ayerst was helping to fund the meeting. They didn't say, "You can't have Dr. Barrett-Connor because we don't like her anymore." Of course not. What they said was, "Oh, this panel isn't bal-anced—it needs a woman gynecologist. How about substituting Dr. X for Barrett-Connor?"

I shouldn't have been surprised. Back in 1994, I wrote in my intro-duction to Sandra Coney's fine book *The Menopause Industry*:

> In the sixties, seventies, and eighties most discussions of
> menopause permitted several points of view. At one extreme were
> the evangelistic proponents such as Robert Wilson. . . . In the

center were those who believed that estrogen might be beneficial for many or most women but that some conditions precluded it: cancer, blood clots, high blood pressure, and perhaps fibroids and gallbladder disease. Lastly in the conservative corner were believers that hormones should be prescribed only for the relief of significant symptoms and with rare exceptions should be reserved for short term use of less than two years. In the 1990 edition of an esteemed reference work, *Goodman and Gilman's the Pharmacological Basis of Therapeutics* was still stating, "The routine prophylactic use of estrogen is difficult to justify. . . . When used, estrogens should be administered in the lowest effective dose for the shortest possible time."

Those two sentences express the essence of the conservative view, but by the next edition, in the mid-nineties, even Goodman and Gilman had joined the estrogen stampede. Although there were no important new clinical studies, somehow, as a result of pharmaceutical tentacles that seemed to reach everywhere—peer review panels at the finest medical journals determining what got published, advisory committees at the NIH deciding whose research got funded, FDA panels determining what drugs were approved, medical-school tenure committees controlling academic physicians' careers and continuing medical education—there was zero tolerance for the conservative position on any estrogen product, including birth control pills. The conservative view was no longer admitted on talk shows and rarely seen in magazines or newspapers that take drug advertising. The elimination of the conservative position from the public view had been hastened by the change in rules that prescription drugs could now be advertised directly to the consumer, which increased the industry's media clout. As I concluded in my 1994 introduction, "That long-term hormone treatment is still experimental, still controversial, still considered dangerous by more than a few authorities is concealed from general viewers and readers. In the nineties I have given interviews to scores of magazine writers only to have my comments removed from the final copy. In the nineties I have been called by and booked on all three network morning programs, only to be canceled out with some lame excuse."

But I was a reporter, not on the cutting edge of research like Dr. Barrett-Connor or Dr. Susan Love, who both were widely admired. I was flabbergasted when *The New York Times* as well as *The New Yorker* attacked Dr. Love's superb 1997 *Hormone Book*. Happily, *The New Yorker*'s talented science writer Malcolm Gladwell, author of "The Estrogen Question: How Wrong Is Dr. Susan Love?" has apologized to her. Here is a bit from their correspondence:

Dear Dr. Love,

You are very right to write to me so thoughtfully and civilly after the article I wrote about you. You were right, and I was wrong, and I apologize for being so dismissive. I have learned my lesson. Science is fickle, and one should never pretend to know anything with certainty. . . . Cheers—and all the best with your work.

Malcolm Gladwell

I was also flabbergasted when, in 1988, after being invited to speak at a gynecologist meeting, Love was openly attacked, on a personal level, by Dr. Charles Hammond, the heavyweight author of CME courses for

Wyeth. He accused her of "believing in herbs" and stated that he regretted the $17 he spent on her book. Hammond did not apologize but many doctors in the audience did.

WYETH GETS ITS COMEUPPANCE

October 3, 2002, was a bleak day in the history of the company now called Wyeth. It had been on credit watch for a week, and on this morning its rating outlook was moved to negative due to its approximately $10 billion in outstanding debt. Revenues from the Premarin family of products, including Prempro, had declined by 25 percent. Wyeth was also having its share of class-action lawsuits from its vaccines and its contraceptive Norplant, by now discontinued. But its greatest disaster was Fen-Phen, the diet drug almost entirely marketed to women that was pulled from drugstore shelves in September 1997 amid scandalous reports that famed obesity experts, such as the University of Pennsylvania's Dr. Albert Stunkard, had signed their names to medical articles that were prepared and paid for by Wyeth. Bringing the matter up to date five years later, Reuters explained:

> Wyeth, formerly known as American Home Products, in recent years had to pay billions of dollars to former users of two diet drugs once included in the "fen-phen" slimming cocktail, to settle lawsuits alleging the drugs caused heart damage. Chief Financial Officer Kenneth Martin told analysts and investors on a conference call Friday that "Wyeth will take an additional reserve of $1.4 billion in addition to the $13.2 billion the firm has already taken to cover litigation" . . . adding "possible additional reserves may be required."

But if the company uses strong-arm tactics against its critics, so, in a very different fashion, do some of the lawyers who stand up for injured patients. I don't know whether these women "earn" their settlements more for the medical hell they go through or for the legal. We mainly hear about Fen-Phen cases because the losses are so staggering, but Wyeth is awash with other lawsuits as well. In the summer of 2002, however, they had one piece of luck, emerging victorious (along with Schering and Organon) in a class-action suit brought by more than a hundred Englishwomen for the failure to warn of an increased risk of blood clots in third-generation oral contraceptives (low-dose pills containing newer progestins such as deso-gestrel and gestodene).

No sooner was the Prempro trial halted than scores of malpractice attorneys posted their shingles on the Internet. Among the first to check them out was Judith Raphael Kletter, who had a mini-stroke—a transient ischemic attack (TIA)—on December 26, 1998, after she had been on Prempro for six months. Kletter was fifty-four years old, a professional researcher who worked for many years at the *International Reader's Digest* procuring obscure artwork and photographs from all over the world. She never felt she needed hormones, but "after reading articles, listening to the news and doctors I thought I would be foolish not to jump on the band-wagon." Her TIA occurred as she was "sitting in my car in Manchester, Vermont, waiting for my husband, Michael, to come out of the hardware store. I was reading storefront signs and suddenly realized I could not focus on the first few letters. I kept blinking but this did not help. A few minutes later, when I regained vision in my left eye, I noticed that I was seeing multiple letters that were precisely symmetrical. I ignored this inci-dent, and a few minutes later I noticed that a black curtain was starting to come down over my eyes." Kletter thought she might have a torn retina, but her doctor sent her for a neurological workup and the stroke was confirmed. In her words, she considers herself "fortunate that I do not have cancer. [But] since my TIA, I live in fear that I will have a major stroke. I have to take blood thinners daily and I was denied long-term health-care insurance."

Kletter joined a class-action lawsuit, but locating an attorney who seemed informed and respectful was no easy task. She finally selected a law firm that treated her with courtesy and respect, and was "interested in short-term effects as well as long, for the side effects of short-term usage can be just as detrimental as long-term." Kletter had quickly gathered that some lawyers are ignorant of the fact that, while the greater risk of cancer weighs in after four or five years, the heart attacks, blood clots, and strokes may start to occur as early as the first few months. "Some law firms are handling only cancer victims, while others are looking for unusual side effects," she further notes. The firm she chose accepted her as a client without pressing her to send them "mountains of medical records." As Kletter says:

> After reading the WHI report in the July 2002 issue of the *Journal of the American Medical Association*, I frequented the World Wide Web to learn everything I could. I began tracking all the class action law firms that appeared looking for victims of Prempro. I immediately began questioning their motivation and concern, asking what their allegation was, what their screening processes entailed, and what types of victims they were looking for. The responses I've received to my questions have been quite interesting and the questionnaire/litigation retainer agreement packets I've been receiving are varied in size and content. Most law firms seem to be requesting up front lots of forms from drugstores, doctors, hospitals, and so forth before they decide to accept their clients. This method leads to a great deal of research and stress on the part of the victims, only to be told by many law

firms, when they receive their information, that they will not accept them as clients. Amazingly, some law firms I called were clueless in knowing what direction they are planning to take. The majority didn't have a clue what their allegations were but just put their names on the Internet looking for victims without having a cause of action.

This state of affairs is inexcusable. Many injured women were bullied by their doctors into taking estrogen that they didn't want or need to "protect" their health. Now they are subjected to being bullied and intimidated by lawyers who also may not know what they are doing. Still, once the more capable and compassionate attorneys rise to the surface, these class-action suits just might turn out to be bigger than the litigation over Fen-Phen—perhaps second only to the cases against the tobacco industry, since so many millions of women have taken Premarin and so many thousands have been harmed. I do not deny that many women are certain that their quality of life has been enhanced by hormones, but most of these are women who needed them and asked for them, not those who were persuaded by false theories of long-term prevention.

WHY DOCTORS REMAIN COY

However well-meaning the doctors may have been, I hope that the lawsuits will make them more cautious and that they will stop prescribing approved drugs for unapproved uses. Let me recap. The FDA never accepted Wyeth's plea to list heart-disease prevention as a reason to prescribe Premarin. Indeed, a key moment that determined the Women's Health Initiative clinical trials occurred in 1990, when Cindy Pearson of the National

Women's Health Network urged the FDA to withhold approval until the right kind of research could be done. The moment of truth came when Pearson pointed out that no drug was ever approved for cardio protection in males unless it was verified by clinical trials, using placebos as a control. What's sauce for the goose and so forth. The FDA staffers at that meeting were convinced.

Are the doctors as responsible as the drug industry? In some situations, they are more so. The responsibility of drug-company officials is to their shareholders and employees, while the gynecologist's responsibility is to the patient. "One law firm," Kletter recalls, "even said that the doctors were the victims as much as the women were because they were misled by Wyeth. I wrote that law firm a nasty letter," she added.

Here is how I see the culpability of doctors: If a woman suffered from symptoms of menopause or had had her ovaries removed or had unexplained fractures in her vertebrae or bones, her doctor would have been correct in prescribing estrogen according to the tenets and scientific findings of the FDA. Not that the FDA is perfect, but the majority of specialists there make every effort to stay on top of ongoing research, adding new indications for drugs when quality research warrants it or deleting them if the drug proves unsafe or is not working as well as had been thought.

But prevention or treatment of heart disease and Alzheimer's with estrogen was never approved by the FDA, for no conclusive studies had shown that the drug worked in those areas. Doctors who prescribed Premarin for these purposes were overreaching, and their role in any estrogen misadventure warrants consideration. To prescribe an approved drug for a use that the FDA does not consider established is always chancy, but to give a known carcinogen and blood-clot enhancer to a healthy person who has no need of it for symptoms is in my opinion reckless. A related reason for the harm that estrogen has done is that patients could not always avail themselves of the same information that doctors had. Doctors knew, or should have known, that Premarin wasn't approved for heart or memory, but these facts were harder for patients to come by, and, sad to say, it was the medical organizations themselves that lobbied to "protect" patients from the facts.

THE HIDDEN SECRETS OF OFF-LABEL PRESCRIPTIONS

There are two things about medical practice that I didn't learn until middle age—both of them disturbing, both of them brought center stage by the halting of the WHI trial. I know I may be wrong. Certainly I may be overstating these matters, but I promise there is at least a nugget of truth here that you may someday find useful.

The first issue has to do with the question of who has the real science, and the answer struck me as a bolt of lightning on February 14, 1996, at ten A.M. I was at an FDA workshop designed to present a consumer perspective on what sort of information we would like to get with prescription drugs. Dr. David Kessler, the commissioner, opened the meeting, declaring that "we will not rest until consumers get good patient information." Our workshop would continue for two days and Kessler hoped for lots of lively interaction among patients, doctors, nurses, pharmacists, and other specialists, as well as industry advocates such as John Gans of the American Pharmaceutical Association and some kind, lovely people who were there to express their "literacy concerns." (They were representing the rights of people who cannot read or write due to language barriers or physical or mental handicaps.)

Cindy Pearson and I appeared first, speaking for the National Women's Health Network. We were given the opening spot because of the historical position of our organization, which was the first to get patient-information leaflets included with any prescription drug—the birth control pill in 1970. We said the things we always say: that patients deserve to know everything their doctors know, stated in plain language; that patient information should begin (like the labeling for doctors) with a complete checklist of the conditions for which the drug is proved effective; that patients need instructions on when and how to take their meds and what interactions with other drugs and foods to watch out for; that potentially dangerous complications should be highlighted and distinguished from minor side effects. Initially, back in 1970, we asked that the patient-information leaflets be made available in Spanish as well as English. As the years passed we called for translation into other languages as well.

The second speaker was Dr. Roy Schwarz of the AMA. Since Kessler said he was all for lively interaction, I asked Schwarz a question that had troubled me for twenty-six years: "Why is the AMA opposed to giving patients comprehensive information?"

"Not everyone wants it," Schwarz replied.

"Not everyone has to read it. What about those who want to?"

"Those leaflets could undermine the physician-patient relationship."

"But how? Didn't the warnings [that came with] the birth control pill save lives? Women now knew the signs of a blood clot. They knew to stop the pill and get help. Clotting-related deaths from the pill declined as soon as the patients got those warnings."

"That's true. I don't deny it," said Dr. Schwarz.

"Malpractice suits also declined. The patient was forewarned, so the doctor had less liability," I continued.

"Yes, I don't deny that either."

"Please explain. If patient leaflets can save lives and reduce malpractice lawsuits, why is the AMA against them?"

The entire audience of FDA personnel, health professionals, consumer advocates, and a member or two of Congress looked at the doctor expectantly.

"It's because of the off-label prescribing," Schwarz declared, looking embarrassed or maybe apologetic.

"What do you mean?"

"Off-label. We think that almost half of prescriptions are written for conditions where the doctor thinks they work but the FDA hasn't approved them [for such purposes]. That's where it would interfere with our relationships. The patient would look at the paper and say, 'He wasn't supposed to prescribe it for this.'"

I was astounded. "Do you mean that the doctors are afraid that if the patients get accurate labeling they will think their doctors are *dumb*?"

He nodded, and then someone else pointed out that if something goes wrong and the drug was prescribed off-label, and if the patient knows it, she is more likely to sue.

A lot of argument was going on around the room, and even others from Schwarz's side of the aisle seemed to be chastising him. But I want him to know that I will always be grateful for the education he gave me that day. And I still think about all those women who didn't quite believe in Premarin for protecting their hearts but whose doctors had hustled them into taking it as so-called preventive medicine.

The lesson I came away with from that workshop was that while doctors might know the real science, they don't want to have to practice it to the letter. They want the right to be creative, to practice intuitively. Half of what they prescribe is no more evidence-based than your grandmother's chicken soup, or maybe even less.

Some reporters at the FDA workshop took their own jabs at the

AMA. A headline on Lauran Neergaard's story for the Associated Press read: "Pharmacists, doctors oppose rule to attach warnings to risky drugs." A second headline, on the "Our View" editorial in USA *Today*, read: "The FDA wants consumers to have more information on drugs. What took so long?"

I might have guessed that the AMA would want to do a little something to get even-steven. Out of the blue, on July 10, 1996, five months after my mano-a-mano with Schwarz at the FDA workshop and twenty-seven years after the fact, *JAMA* published a review of my 1969 book, *The Doctors' Case Against the Pill*—a book that had helped stir public opinion in favor of accurate patient information.

Can you guess what the AMA thought of my old book? They didn't like it. They didn't like it a lot! The reviewer, Dr. Carl J. Levinson, chief of an endoscopic surgery laboratory supported by Ethicon, a division of Johnson & Johnson, which owns Ortho, the world's largest manufacturer of birth control pills, began by stating: "This is a strange book and not particularly recommended." He closed with, "I cannot, in all good conscience, recommend it for either the public or the profession." And those were the nicest things he said.

I can boast that *JAMA* gave me one of the worst reviews I have ever seen in my life, not just of my book but of any book I've ever read a review of. Not only did Levinson have a financial conflict of interest that should have disqualified him from reviewing *The Doctors' Case Against the Pill* (Ortho and Ethicon were listed that year in Johnson & Johnson's annual report as associates in the same women's health marketing division), but he'd recently had a disciplinary action and a reprimand on his California and New York medical licenses for "overprescribing or misprescribing drugs." (He was ordered to take a remedial course in drug prescribing as a condition of keeping those licenses.) Dr. Levinson is also listed in the 2000 edition of *Questionable Doctors Disciplined by State and Federal Governments*.

I didn't get it until later, but I had dealt the bad guys at the AMA a severe blow when I outed their dirty, unscientific secret at that FDA workshop. I was like Toto, pulling aside the curtain behind which was a small, frightened man pretending to be a wizard. To thwart such a wizard, we must *demand* drug information that separates fact from myth, that states clearly and specifically what the drug is approved for so that we don't become unwitting participants in unacknowledged experiments. We also need the "what for" information as a safeguard to recognize the accidental prescription for a wrong drug with a similar name.

Dr. M. Roy Schwarz has left the American Medical Association and is now president of the China Medical Board of New York, a private foundation founded in 1914 to promote high-quality Western medicine in China as well as Thailand, Myanmar, Vietnam, Mongolia, and Nepal. An authority in innovative medical education, he still holds old-fashioned ideals on the doctor-patient relationship, which he sees as a sacred trust. He is still not for patient-information leaflets because he believes a good doctor will explain everything, and perhaps he also believes there are more good doctors than there really are . . . or at least that doctors have more face time with each patient than they actually do. We differ, but I will always respect Dr. Schwarz for divulging the secret that had so long eluded me, and the fact that he did so, flying in the face of his perturbed colleagues, shows how deeply felt is his confidence in the judgment and sincerity of the typical M.D. Yet in October 2002, as we concluded a long conversation, he made a surprising remark:

"An off-label drug for short-term use for symptoms is one thing, but long-term use for prevention is something else. In that case, I would make an exception and take the same side as you. If a woman is going to be taking estrogen to prevent heart disease . . . I wouldn't tell her that it's off-label exactly, but I would want her to know that this application is still under study. Yes, under study, that would be the right term."

Why Oh Why Oh, Wyeth

The second thing I didn't learn about medical practice until I was middle-aged is that what with the off-label use of prescription drugs and spotty quality control in some drug houses, we cannot necessarily count on traditional prescription and OTC drugs to be more "scientific" or reliable than alternatives. Think for a moment and compare. What if all the people taking ginkgo biloba to enhance their memories were informed that "a great study proves it doesn't work at all. In fact, it might make your memory worse." Some might be disappointed or curse themselves for throwing away money, but devastated, distraught, deeply puzzled and confused—I don't think so. When we try alternative medicines, it's with hope and an open mind, but we are not *counting* on them. Indeed, we take it as an article of faith that these products have been nowhere near so scientifically studied and tested as our prescription drugs.

Now suppose there was a second great ginkgo biloba study, and this time we were told: "Ginkgo will improve your short-term memory by 50 percent. But it must be ginkgo from a certain section of China, picked only in certain seasons, and freeze-dried." Some of us would believe that, too, and we might give Chinese ginkgo a chance. We might say, "Well, it's plausible because, unlike prescription drugs, alternative treatments lack uniform standards. When one fails, you might luck into another brand that works."

Well, I am here to tell you that the same holds true for some FDA-regulated drugs, those sold over-the-counter as well as those available by prescription only. It wasn't until I got interested in the disappearance of the Today sponge and began digging deep into some not-for-public-consumption archives at the FDA that I saw the extent to which quality control can fail, which is not to say that there is *no* difference in the reliability of regulated and unregulated products. There is a difference indeed, but it's not absolute. While the FDA does its best to protect our drug supply, certain companies have repeated and ongoing problems with quality control. Wyeth is one of them. We cannot count on the quality of all their products, prescription or over-the-counter, to outrank the better brands of alternative medicines.

By way of explanation, let me take you back to 1994, when I heard from several readers that they were unable to buy the Today-brand contraceptive sponge, a nonhormonal barrier product with a small but loyal following, because they were out of stock and pharmacists were unable to determine why. When I checked on the situation, I found the manufacturer (an affiliate of Wyeth) evasive, and at first the FDA as well, but on January 12, 1995, the FDA's Donald C. McLearn wrote the following:

> The Today Sponge has been in short supply since the firm stopped production after FDA's inspection in March 1994 of the only facility manufacturing the contraceptive.
>
> The comprehensive inspection of the firm's plant in Hammonton, N.J., disclosed bacterial contamination of the water used to make the Today Sponge as well as other products manufactured in the facility, including nasal sprays, ointments and suppositories.
>
> FDA investigators also established that the firm had neglected to validate its microbiological test methods, thereby raising

questions about their reliability. Still other problems were found in the firm's equipment sanitization.

Recently, after weighing the cost of modifications that would be necessary to bring the Hammonton plant up to acceptable manufacturing standards, as well as the likely loss of Today Sponge's market share by the time the upgrading would be completed, the firm announced its decision to stop making the contraceptive.

The agency did not object to continued production of Today Sponge under appropriate manufacturing and hygienic conditions. Long-standing public health standards, however, do not allow the marketing of contaminated products that present a potential risk of disease transmission.

At first, I thought that the Today sponge was just a bad apple on the Hammonton tree, but on further investigation, I found a "Warning Letter" dated March 19, 1993, from the FDA to Mr. Stanley Barchey, chief executive officer of Whitehall Laboratories Division of American Home Products.

Dear Mr. Barchey,

During an inspection of Whitehall Laboratories, on February 3–March 1, 1993, located at 1000 South Grand Street, Hammonton, New Jersey, our investigator documented serious violations of the Food, Drug and Cosmetic Act with respect to Current Good Manufacturing Practices as set forth under Title 21, Code of Federal Regulations . . . involving the manufacture, processing, packaging, testing and distribution of Advil Tablets, Dristan Gel Capsules, Anacin Tablets, Maximum Strength

Anacin Tablets, Arthritis Pain Formula Caplets, Preparation H
Suppositories and Today Contraceptive Sponge. . . .

What followed was a single-spaced six-page letter signed by Matthew H. Lewis of the FDA's Mid-Atlantic Region office in West Orange, New Jersey. Here is a sampling of the violations (note that they refer to specific batches tested and may or may not apply more widely):

- Preparation H ointment "was noted to be contaminated with isopropyl alcohol from the cleaning lines."
- Preparation H suppositories failed the codes for content uniformity. For example, "the product failed the specification for Shark Liver Oil."
- Dristan Gel caplets failed specifications for content uniformity.
- Sleep-eze tablets, Batch H-1 rejected for possible metal contamination.
- Yeast mold was noted in the raw materials for Aspirin-Free Anacin.
- Foreign matter was discovered in Arthritis Pain Formula. The foreign matter was caused by a "vertical feed screw" coming loose and eroding a belt located directly above the Chilsonator, where the product enters the mill. The design of the Chilsonator was found to be inadequate to prevent foreign matter from contaminating the batch.
- Packaging date codes for Advil were inaccurate. Stability batches revealed that packaging date codes are not truly representative of the product age.

- Dristan failed analysis for pseudoephedrine and brompheniramine maleate.
- The investigation conducted into the consumer complaint for Today Sponge was grossly inadequate in that the investigation report stated the consumer reported two torn sponges. This report further states that the "Line logs for this batch show no molding problems." However, it was noted that 15 percent of the batch (65,526 sponges) was rejected for product failures.

As time passed, the FDA made it known that Hammonton was by no means the company's only substandard plant. In 1995, the FDA cited serious violations at Wyeth-Ayerst factories in Marietta, Pennsylvania, and Pearl River, New York. The agency assured consumers it never found contaminated products and was aware of no illnesses arising from them, but that the manufacturing problems constituted "serious violations of rules meant to ensure that drugs and vaccines are sterile and of high quality."

Amazing as it may seem, five years after the violations had been discovered, they still were not satisfactorily corrected. Among the products manufactured at these factories were flu vaccines, and in the fall of 2000, the vaccine failed FDA safety tests. Production was halted until the problems could be fixed, and the disruption contributed to a national emergency. Health officials were forced to prioritize the available supply, ordering that the first available flu shots be reserved for the elderly and chronically ill. The company's noncompliant practices resulted in big news and a fat fine. Wyeth-Ayerst agreed to pay $30 million for its repeated violations and a former FDA official who had joined Wyeth acknowledged to an AP reporter that "Thirty million dollars is substantial money to us, no doubt about that. It is clear that the FDA did regard these problems as problems that needed more attention and a faster pace than we achieved."

Nor, as we now know, did Wyeth's problems begin or end there. Take Norplant, marketed in the United States in 1990 as a long-acting (five-year) hormonal contraceptive wherein small rods containing a pro-gestin called levonorgestrel are implanted in a woman's arm. Prior to the drug's approval, women's rights activists feared that it would be used coer-cively on low-income women. Inspired by Belita Cowan's exposé of flawed research on morning-after pills (see chapter 5), these activists located women who'd participated in pre-market clinical trials in Europe, Asia, and Brazil, and compared what they had to say about their Norplant expe-riences with what the researchers published. Yes, there were women who liked Norplant and adjusted well, but the majority had some complaints. Many had unpredictable and lengthy menstrual periods, which proved a hardship for religious Muslims and Orthodox Jews because according to strict practices in both faiths, a menstruating woman can't participate in sexual intercourse. Then there were the prostitutes in Thailand who brought a loss-of-income lawsuit, as they could not perform their job. Many of the Norplant providers stuck to a position that the bleeding might clear up on its own and posed no danger. They refused to remove the rods. However, the most bitter of the trial veterans were those who had suffered injuries when doctors did attempt removal. In one out of every five or six users, the rods migrated or broke, and the surgery got dicey.

The National Women's Health Network asked the FDA to defer approval of Norplant until Wyeth agreed to provide consent forms warning of the problems and promised to remove the rods free of charge at the patient's request. The FDA's Dr. Philip Corfman asked further that the manufacturer provide special training in rod-removal techniques. But instead of agreeing to present Norplant with safety measures in place, the company and the nonprofit Population Council that had developed the device staged an attack on the health activists, charging that according to an article in the December 16, 1990, *New York Times Sunday Magazine,* their standards were "too high," and adding that it was not the lawyers and their injury suits that had halted contraceptive research but picky consumers.

Soon there *were* lawsuits, the contraceptive got a bad reputation, and sales became disappointing. Then, in the summer of 2000, the corporate bugaboo of flaws in the manufacture struck Norplant. Letters went to health professionals advising that the lots distributed in 1999 with expiration dates in 2004 had "atypically low levels of levonorgestrel release in routine shelf-life stability tests." Patients should be warned to use backup contraception for the time being. Two years later, on July 26, 2002, doctors and patients were informed that "after further evaluation, FDA and Wyeth have determined that patients do not need to use any backup nonhormonal method of birth control." However, Wyeth also decided that "due to limitations in component supplies, the company would no longer distribute the six-implant system."

And so for the last two years of Norplant's twelve-year U.S. life span, women who were on the drug had to use a second contraceptive as well, only to be told they hadn't needed the extra birth control after all and that Norplant was being withdrawn. In my view, Wyeth might have spared itself the lawsuits and the outrage of women if they had honestly told these patients what to expect.

Now let's look at Provera, truly a wild card, the "pro" in Prempro. In July 2002, farmers throughout Europe rose up to threaten lawsuits against Wyeth's Irish affiliate, Elan. The charge: Animal feed shipped from

Ireland for their cows and pigs was contaminated with Provera. Residues of the hormone were found in the animals, which made them unsuitable for the European food supply, where hormones are outlawed. According to news reports, some of the farmers were beside themselves; a full year's income or more might be at stake. I asked the FDA's Dr. Lisa Rarick, who has a background in hormone products (indeed, she was FDA project officer, under Dr. Corfman, on the approval of Norplant), if she'd guess how the Irish Provera got so misappropriated. She speculated that it might be a result of "either the mislabeling of the water or mishandling of the waste."

Now we come to Wyeth's ace-in-the hole, the hormone Premarin. The year 2001 was a bounty year for Premarin profits. As noted, if you add in Prempro and do the math, the Premarin family of drugs retained its number one position. More than that, profits were increased by radically raising prices. A report revealed that the cost of the fifty drugs most prescribed for seniors rose by an average of nearly three times the rate of inflation. But Premarin was one of only three drugs to get away with through-the-roof price hikes, at seven times the inflation rate.

Yet while the Premarin coffers were filling up fast, Wyeth failed to complete a long-standing recall of pills that don't dissolve at the proper rate. Is this dangerous? Probably not, although it's conceivable that extra large bursts of estrogen might provoke a blood clot in women who are vulnerable. More likely, if the patient is getting too little Premarin in her pill, hot flashes might recur; if too much, the result can be sore breasts and nausea. Dr. Rogerio Lobo, a respected gynecologist at Columbia University but also a paid researcher and advocate for Premarin, assured the public that no harm was possible. When I called and e-mailed him to ask on what he based his conclusion, he never got back to me.

This particular Premarin problem may have been cloaked in some secrecy by the FDA as well as the manufacturer. The FDA, for example, has been slow to pass dissolution information on to the public. Recall letters dated February 21, 2002, were not posted until June 12. Not only that, the recalls were issued by lot numbers, but it's my understanding that such numbers apply only to the large dispensing bottles and usually are not transferred to the retail level, where only the prescribed dosage of pills is given to the patient in small containers.

By 2000, the recall of the faulty Premarin covered some 382 million doses, equivalent to about 17 percent of tablets sold in 1999, according to an on-line article in Thestreet.com. Philip De Vane, American Home's vice president of clinical affairs, refused to discuss the nature of the problem when he was questioned by reporters. However, he maintained that the way compounds dissolve in lab tests "doesn't affect how the drug dissolves in women's bodies." But scientists and stock analysts who specialize in pharmaceuticals aren't so sure. Stefan Loren of Legg Mason, who has a background in both arenas, said: "If the FDA felt the need to have a recall on this scale, I have to believe they felt there was some sort of problem. Perhaps it was relatively minor, but they felt there was risk. You obviously want a medication to have optimal performance and don't want hormone levels to vary in a person's body."

The earliest recall notice that I hold in my hand as I write this is dated January 1999. The most recent is August 2002. The ongoing Premarin recall has been in effect for almost four years. The pills have expiration dates that run through the end of 2003.

A Safety Alert from the FDA dated January 2001 notes that 108,394 bottles with recall numbers had been distributed at that time! The technical name for the procedure is a quality assurance recall. The official reason is that "Testing has revealed the lots do not conform to the USP dissolution specifications for conjugated estrogen tablets."

CHAPTER 7

MADELINE GRAY: WHEN NATURE THROWS THE BOOK AT THE MENOPAUSAL WOMAN

Instead of making you skip the changing years, removing both
ovaries does the opposite. It brings them on with a bang.

— MADELINE GRAY

Hard times can bring out great achievements, as the story of Made-
line Gray illustrates. In 1946, four years after Premarin came on the U.S.
market, Gray had a total hysterectomy, was plunged into a wretched
menopause, got no help from her doctors, heard about Premarin from her
girlfriends, and "found blessed relief. . . . I learned," she said, "that prolonged menopausal suffering is almost unnecessary, since there is now, for
the first time in history, blessed menopausal medicine to help. Our mothers may have had to suffer, not us. We are the first generation lucky
enough to have this help."

But there was a hitch. No one could promise Gray that it was safe to
stay on Premarin for life. Regretting that she'd consented to her hysterectomy,

she vowed to avoid a second mistake. As a journalist, she decided to research the facts for herself and write a report to women as if she were "talking to a friend." The trouble was, she had no credentials: Her previous books included a children's story and two volumes on the restaurant business. But an editor at Doubleday decided to take a flier on Gray and give her a chance. The rest—no exaggeration—is history.

The Changing Years, originally published in 1951, became a best-seller and then a standard, which Gray updated from time to time. Many of Gray's original comments are almost interchangeable with those made some half a century later by Dr. Jacques Rossouw, director of the Women's Health Initiative, and with the international position paper titled *Women's Health and Menopause: A Comprehensive Approach* that he and his colleagues at NIH prepared. For example, much as she loved what Premarin did for her, Gray cautioned: "Take no more estrogen than you need and give it up as quickly as you can. All drugs taken in excess can be harmful. Estrogen can be particularly bad because it is so stimulating. In fact it can be highly overstimulating to the point where it causes all kinds of unwanted results. All menopausal medicine is 'tideover' medicine, not 'cure' medicine. You don't need to cure the menopause because it is not a disease. So the minute you comfortably can, get away from every form of outside help and give your own body the chance to follow through."

Roger Kahn, the sportswriter, whose mother, Olga, was Madeline Groggins Gray's Cornell classmate and lifelong friend, recalls Gray as "short and aggressive, with a sense of humor and a distinctive, throaty voice." Indeed, she was tiny, no more than four feet, ten inches, and her baritone voice was a souvenir—one might say a war wound—from the time she experimented with hormone products on herself and had an unfortunate response to the testosterone wafers she placed under her tongue.

How Her Doctor Dismissed Her
in the Hospital

Gray's odyssey began in her forties when, not yet menopausal, her doctor, a "surgeon with a princely air," detected a fibroid in her uterus and informed her that "we'd better take it out." Back in her hospital room after her surgery, Gray learned that her doctor had removed her ovaries as well. She asked him why, and as if she had no business questioning him, he replied brusquely: "To prevent cancer. You signed the permission form! Did you expect me to wake you up in the middle of the operation for a cup of tea and a cozy chat?"

How Her Doctor Dissed Her Back at Home

Gray had fears that she would "grow a mustache and gain forty pounds," but apprehensions about changes in appearance aside, she felt that biologically "nature threw the book" at her. An average hot flash is over in thirty seconds, but Gray had some that lasted more than ten minutes. Again she tried to question her doctor, "who was both far too busy and too abrupt to bother with me. As to my future worries, he curtly dismissed them by telling me to go home and forget about the whole thing. Besides, the worries were all imaginary anyway."

I was astonished by my first migraine a short time after my menopause started. I had practically never had a headache in my life, but I awoke one morning with this strange, terrible throbbing. I could barely make it from the bed to the bathroom. The light hurt my eyes, so I had to put on dark glasses. I had absolutely no desire to eat. When it lasted three days, getting progressively worse, I was really stumped. At last it dawned on me that it must have something to do with the operation that had brought on my sudden menopause. So I staggered to the phone and called the surgeon. I must have called him at an off minute, for he merely barked, "Nonsense, it has nothing to do with the operation," and abruptly hung up. With my surgeon ruled out as a source of information I next tried questioning friends.

TAKING HER HEALTH IN HER OWN HANDS

Gray read every research paper on estrogen she could find. She wrote to the doctors whose work impressed her and asked them for interviews. She crisscrossed the United States and Canada, visiting clinics, talking with nurses, research scientists, and patients, as well as physicians in diverse specialties. Gray chronicles the miseries that some women have: great waves of heat spreading clear up over the body to the top of the head; drenching sweats; hearts beating so loud that it seems the whole world can hear the sound; fatigue so profound they can hardly move; migraine headaches that seem like "brain pains"; pain in the back of the neck; pains in the chest characteristic of a heart attack; pains in the joints that seem like arthritis; irritability; tension; depression. But however bad the symptoms, over time most of the patients she interviewed were able to give up the "tideover" medicine. It took novelist Faith Baldwin eight years, but Gray herself, more typically, returned to normal after three years. Some lucky women recovered in weeks or months. In fact, Gray learned that the majority of women experienced menopause as no big deal. According to her research, only one in four felt so symptomatic as to ask for hormone supplements.

And those like Gray, who'd had their ovaries removed, tended to have the most discomfort.

One of Gray's discoveries was that many patients were discouraged from following their own preferences. A woman might be fit and symptom-free, but if her doctor believed in estrogen, she was expected to take it. That situation hasn't changed until very recently. One of my neighbors told me she'd been on estrogen for fifteen years, but on the day she heard about the halted study she threw out her pills. I asked how she was feeling. "Fine," she said. "No difference. No better and no worse." I asked her why she took the drug. She said she didn't know—only that, following her final menstruation, the doctor gave her a prescription.

"But why did you stay on it?" I asked.

She shrugged: "Two words: *in irtia*."

At the other extreme, doctors who *didn't* believe in estrogen often withheld it from their most menopausally miserable patients. It's all about the doctor, as if it were an article of faith, having little to do with either the science or the needs of the patient at hand. Then as now, the doctor's ego may be paramount. Thirty years after Gray brought up the subject in the initial publication of *The Changing Years*, Dr. Robert Mendelsohn, chairman of the Illinois State Medical Licensing Committee and therefore privy to frequent complaints of malpractice, wrote his own exposé: *MalePractice: How Doctors Manipulate Women*. He warned readers to watch out for doctors who use clichés such as the following:

- "Trust me, dear"
- "It's a good thing you came to see me when you did"
- "What medical school did *you* go to?"
- "There, there, dear, don't worry your pretty little head"

- "Take these and you'll feel better"
- "What do you need a uterus for, anyway?"
- "It's safer than pregnancy"
- "You'll be okay. Just leave everything to me"
- "I'm going to sew you up like a virgin"
- "Your pelvis is too small"
- "You'll just have to learn to live with it"

Dr. Alan Guttmacher, the late president of Planned Parenthood, deeply opposed to unnecessary surgery and therefore in the same corner as Mendelsohn and Gray, coauthored a famous study for the Teamsters Union showing when the members got health insurance, their wives were hustled into getting hysterectomies, of which 40 percent turned out to be unnecessary or questionable. Some called these operations "hip-pocket hysterectomies," in the belief that the only beneficiary was the doctor's wallet. I asked Dr. Guttmacher if the term was justified, and he said it was more complicated than that. "Don't forget that gynecologists are surgeons," he explained. "Generals are trained to fight and they want to fight. Surgeons are trained to operate and they want to operate."

Having interviewed women in their seventies who had hot flashes when their ovaries were removed, Madeline Gray insisted that the postmenopausal ovary continued hormone production—a fact, she said, that had been known since 1947. She therefore strongly urged women to keep their healthy ovaries intact and to always seek a second opinion when surgery was suggested. In later editions of *The Changing Years*, Gray added a chapter entitled "Don't Rush into Hysterectomy." She wrote that the risk of ovarian cancer was less than 30 women per 100,000 per year, while the risk of dying or being seriously harmed by a hysterectomy or the anesthesia involved was higher than that, so removing the ovaries for cancer prevention did not make sense. However, the more sold that gynecologists became on estrogen, the more bent they were on persuading menopausal women to ditch their ovaries, as if the sole purpose of these organs now was to lurk there waiting for cancer to strike.

Gray lived a long and productive life but didn't make it to 1999, much less 2002, the years her research and beliefs were vindicated. In 1999, the American College of Obstetricians and Gynecologists (ACOG) issued a new Practice Bulletin, altering its guidelines. The Bulletin noted that some 600,000 uterine hysterectomies were performed in the United States each year, and that about half of those patients (300,000) agreed to simultaneous oophorectomy. While "preventive removal may be justified in some cases, especially with high risk patients," the guidelines stated, ACOG rescinded its previous recommendation that all women over forty should give up their ovaries along with their uterus. In 2002, as we know, Gray's caution against keeping women on hormones also was proved correct.

Madeline Gray, a bright woman with no medical training, was merely a good listener and a good reporter, and she was right for fifty years while the doctors were wrong. Not that she didn't make mistakes. Brief though it may have been, Gray enjoyed a flirtation with the male hormone. "Androgens are given in much the same ways as estrogen is given—by mouth, by injection, by cream and by pellet. An excellent way is in the form of wafers that dissolve slowly in the mouth like old-fashioned hard candy. If taken in this way practically all the medicine is absorbed directly into the bloodstream instead of some being destroyed as it is worked upon by the stomach secretions, and this seems to give especially good results." According to Gray, "Being the male or 'strength' hormone, it is far better than estrogen in cases of general weakness or fatigue. Also in cases of frigidity or lack of sex desire." I don't know if her self-administered testosterone trial was a mistake per se. Perhaps she accidentally overdosed. Yet despite her voice change, she never seemed to regret the experience.

Gray doesn't come out and say so, but she hints that she may have fiddled with thyroid supplements as well. "Thyroid, along with estrogen and androgen, can still be another comfort while you change. It is a general energy hormone. Sometimes a general push is what you need." Perhaps she needed the thyroid as well as the testosterone to give her the push needed to finish her comprehensive and entertaining book. Certainly she must have read every pertinent publication in the library at the New York Academy of Medicine. I know because there were occasions — thirty, forty, fifty years after she had published *The Changing Years* — when library aides would bring me an early book or scientific paper on hormones or menopause, and I would see that Madeline Gray was the last person, or almost the last, to have checked it out.

The second edition of *The Changing Years* was published in 1958, and the third in 1967, a year after *Feminine Forever*. At the time, Gray delivered Robert Wilson a slap on the wrist, although she had softened somewhat on the long-term use of hormones:

> When I wrote the first edition of this book doctors considered menopausal hormones strictly as "tideover medicine." But recently there has been a change of opinion. Many doctors now believe that menopausal hormones are not tideover medicine but replacement medicine, and continue giving them to some women whether they have symptoms or not. . . . Estrogen, they say, favors the laying down of calcium in the bones. . . . To minimize the possibility of things like osteoporosis, coronary attacks and dizzy spells increasing as time goes by, many doctors are now

giving some of their patients estrogen not only during but long after the menopause. Indeed, they even are giving it to the ripe old age of ninety and more.

So did Madeline Gray go back on Premarin after all? We'll never know, but here is how she dismisses Wilson:

> *Not "pills to keep you young" or "feminine forever."* These doctors [giving long-term hormones], unlike some others, are not going to the extreme of calling estrogen "pills to keep you young." Nor are they claiming they will keep you "feminine forever." For they know there is not a single substance known that can keep you in a state of constant youth—any more than blackstrap molasses can or honey and vinegar . . . in fact falling for far-out fads and promises may only leave you sadder and more disappointed than ever.

If I were a betting woman I would place my money on Gray's not having gone back on hormones, although she may have used vaginal suppositories or creams as needed, for she was very fond of sex. But Gray had read the animal research from the 1930s and '40s, and it was clear that these reports worried her. Here's her verdict on cancer: "Estrogen alone cannot cause cancer in human beings. We don't know what can, but none of the available evidence to date points to estrogen alone. It must be estrogen combined with something else." Even Charlie Dodds or Michael Shimkin—or Jacques Rossouw—might say they agree.

CHAPTER 8

POISON BY PRESCRIPTION

As it turned out, it was an arrogant, overreaching surgeon, an ovary snatcher, whose cruelty and contempt prompted Madeline Gray to undertake her remarkable work. I envy people who go through life having only good experiences with medical care, but I, like Gray, am not among them. In 1957 my son, Noah, was born in Cincinnati. Those were the days when the infant-formula companies convinced doctors that their products were nutritionally superior to mother's milk. Thus my doctor and I had a misunderstanding. I told him I intended to breastfeed. He told me I wouldn't make a good cow. I asked him why. He said I was too educated and excitable. I said I was like my mother and she had breastfed me. I thought that settled the matter, but my doctor was accustomed to having his orders obeyed. He took it upon himself to prescribe a laxative that nursing mothers should never take. My baby lost a third of his birthweight and became perilously ill. He recovered, but in one sense I did not, for I would never again trust a doctor blindly. And then when Noah was a year old, my aunt Sally died from her Premarin-induced cancer.

Healthy baby, healthy aunt, and both of them poisoned by prescription. Going against the tide, I wrote an article on breastfeeding and a cautionary article on menopause treatments. Then, just as America was going crazy for the new birth control pill, I got a call to arms from Dr. Joyce Brothers, the TV psychologist, who hired me as a writer on her advice show. We were swamped with questions and comments on Enovid, the first oral contraceptive. Some viewers were disappointed that it ruined their sex lives, making them feel *toujours* pregnant. Some husbands, on the other hand, wrote in to declare that having had a taste of sex on the pill, they would never again go back to condoms or that "greasy kid stuff." We heard from cautious doctors who recognized that the early pills might be too strong, and from a gynecology professor who insisted that 10,000 volunteers in Puerto Rico took the pill and not one of them ever had a side effect.

As I checked out the science, I was startled to learn how similar the different estrogen products really were once they metabolized in a woman's body. In the hope of avoiding uterine cancer, some doctors were even giving menopausal patients Enovid instead of Premarin. No question, though, all of the hormone products were breaking sales records in the 1960s, the decade when Premarin lifted off thanks to Medicare, Robert Wilson, and Sondra Gorney's Information Center on the Mature Woman. And also the decade in which the pill helped to jump-start a movement for women's rights. Many agreed with playwright Clare Boothe Luce, who declared to a reporter at the *Los Angeles Times*: "With the Pill, modern woman is at last free, as a man is free, to dispose of her own body, to earn her living, to pursue the improvement of her mind, to try a successful career."

In her authoritative 1998 book, *On the Pill: A Social History of Oral Contraceptives*, Dr. Elizabeth Siegel Watkins, a Harvard-trained historian of science, agreed with Luce's assessment, writing:

In spite of the backlash against the pill at the end of the 1960s and continued doubts about its safety through the 1980s, the birth control pill has had an undeniably significant effect on certain segments of the American population. White, middle-class married women who could afford the pill and the private physicians who prescribed them benefited most from oral contraception in the 1960s. The pill offered easy, reliable effective protection against pregnancy, which empowered women to plan when to have children and how many to have.

Watkins added that by 1990, 80 percent of all American women born since 1945 had tried the pill.

Much less recognized in the 1960s, but nonetheless a part of our lives and of the Greatest Experiment, was Charlie Dodds's misbegotten diethylstilbestrol, which held a larger share of the market than any other hormone. It was still prescribed for pregnant women, although the Karnaky/Smith claims that it would prevent miscarriage were never proved. But far more pervasive was its use in animal feed. The treatment of cattle, sheep, and poultry with DES became popular at the end of World War II, and by the 1960s, 80 to 85 percent of our livestock was raised on DES, traces of which were served up to us at the dinner table. The point, of course, was to fatten up livestock so it could be brought to market sooner, cutting feed costs by 10 percent. And bear in mind that in the United States, where pharmacists sell hormones and antibiotics by prescription only, in feed stores you could buy the same products by the carload with no prescription. However, as M. E. Royce, a physician from El Centro, California, protested, "The meat animal on DES retains salt and water in its tissues, even as the lady on birth control pills retains salt and water in her tissues.

All [this] does for the consumer is to cause the meat to splatter in the pan while frying, making it necessary to clean up the stove more often."

Beatrice Trum Hunter, a writer on natural foods and author of an influential book called *Consumer Beware!*, explains, "Stilbestrol yields poorer meat because it produces weight that is watery fat, not protein. From the consumer's point of view this is not only undesirable but also an economic fraud." But there was more at stake than spattered stoves and inflated prices. Dodds himself was worried about the cancer-causing effects of ingested DES, and that was why he favored pellet implants that could be removed before slaughter, with, he thought, less chance of leaving residues in the animal tissues. Even so, the ranchers and poultrymen were often careless. Pellets remaining in chicken necks would frequently surface in soup or be swallowed by restaurant workers, who were frequently served up the spare parts of birds not deemed fit for customer consumption; it was not unusual for such men to grow breasts, just as the workers in Dodds's laboratory did. Also, all the DES-dosed cows and sheep and chickens were excreting tons and tons of waste with hormones in them. Traces were discovered in soil and in waterways. Fish and other creatures were turning hermaphroditic or sterile, leading some scientists to wonder if the waste from DES and other estrogens might be a factor in the rising rates of hormone-dependent cancers in human males.

Then, too, there were the health risks posed to our household pets and other small animals. This came to light when mink ranchers discovered that the feed for their animals, bearing mysterious names such as "digest of chicken by-products and chicken parts," was making them sterile, a condition traced to the remains of undissolved DES pellets. When I heard about this, I checked the labels on my cat-food tins, and sure enough, they contained the same by-products, so I threw them out.

GAYLORD NELSON: "THESE HEARINGS CONCERN YOUR HEALTH AND YOUR POCKETBOOK"

Like Robert Greenblatt, who was the first to advocate testosterone for menopausal women, Gaylord Nelson, an idealistic young lawyer from Clear Lake, Wisconsin, also served in Japan in World War II. An Army captain, he was shipped to Okinawa as a white officer in charge of an all-Negro unit. While Greenblatt investigated the A-bomb damage at Nagasaki, Nelson conducted his own battles to protest the second-class Jim Crow treatment his men received. (When Gaylord Nelson was eight or nine years old, his father, a country doctor, had taken him to hear Robert "Fighting Bob" La Follette, leader of the Progressive Party, speak from the back of a train. The boy instantly embraced La Follette as his idol and threw his cap in the ring for a political life. Young Nelson was still in knee pants when he mounted his first campaign to save the environment by planting trees along the five roads leading into his hometown. And yes, he's the one who would eventually become the Father of Earth Day.)

Robert Greenblatt would spend much of his postwar life exploring new uses for hormones and other drugs. Gaylord Nelson, by contrast, would one day use the power vested in him as a U.S. senator to "expose the pharmaceutical industry to public scrutiny." With his homespun medical background as the son of a doctor, and wed to Carrie Lee Dotson, a nurse, he had an insider's knowledge of the problems in health care and harbored no delusions about the bombast of Big Pharma's claim that its goal was to "help people." He and his wife were viewed by others in Congress with a mixture of awe and disdain because they lived on only his salary. He was said to be the only senator who did so. He was old-fashioned. He represented no one's interests but his constituents'.

In 1967, soon after programs such as Medicaid and Medicare were federally funded, Nelson became chairman of a Senate subcommittee on monopoly. The hearings he was to hold would be "concerned with the important matter of the health and the pocketbook of American citizens," he announced on his opening day. Over a ten-year period, his subcommittee filled thirty Government Printing Office (GPO) volumes, some as thick as 1,500 pages, with incisive exposés on how the drug industry comports itself. He found that pharmaceutical firms often "compromise the quality of new drug evaluations," and he raised the standards. He found that doctors as well as the FDA depended on industry for drug information, which might not be objective since "each company tried to portray its product in the best possible light." He encouraged the FDA to establish a system of independent advisory panels. He exposed the abuse of antibiotics and anti-obesity drugs, the misleading claims for cough and cold remedies and the questionable advertisements for over-the-counter drugs, as well as the seduction of doctors and medical students through lavish gifts. He excoriated the makers of antidepressants for setting ridiculously low standards of who should use them. At one hearing, he quoted an ad for the powerful drug Triavil that suggested a list of questions to ask patients, and he answered the questions himself.

"Lately, have you often felt . . . sad or unhappy? Pessimistic about the future? Disinterested in others? Disappointed in others? Disappointed with yourself? Easily tired?"

. . . I answered all of these yes.

"Have you recently had difficulty making decisions?"

I changed my vote twice in a month on the same issue.

His conclusion: "I think that almost everybody is going to give a yes answer to 70 percent of these questions, so you would end up with everybody on that drug every day."

Thirty years after that episode, antidepressants and tranquilizers are promoted with the selfsame techniques. As I write this, with sales of the Premarin products greatly reduced (Prempro sales were down 40 percent in November 2002; Premarin itself was down 15 percent), Wyeth is trying to take up the slack with an aggressive promotion for Effexor targeted to college students. They are trading in Lauren Hutton, so to speak, for Cara Kahn, a young star of MTV who takes Effexor to treat her own depression. "In accepting the job I really made it clear that I am not a walking commercial," said Kahn in an interview. Yet Wyeth plans to feature her as a spokeswoman at ninety-minute forums in campus auditoriums around the country—programs offering free screenings to inform the audience why they need Effexor. Both Kahn and Wyeth decline to say how much the company is paying her.

When Gaylord Nelson took the Triavil quiz, he did answer "no" to the question asking if he had "difficulty working." To be sure, this senator had energy to spare and a knack for keeping multiple plates spinning in the air. His priorities were a passionate love of nature and an equally passionate obsession with fair play. Therefore in many ways it was in keeping with his lifelong goals that on December 29, 1969, Senator Nelson released a statement to the press in which he announced he had "scheduled hearings to explore the question of whether users of birth control pills are being adequately informed concerning the pill's known health hazards," adding how important it is "that women be informed about all aspects of the use of the pill so that they are able to make an intelligent, personal decision about [its] use." Nelson said oral contraceptives were being relied upon by 8.5 million women in the United States and 10 million elsewhere, and that in British studies of the pill, it had been reported that 1 in every 2,000 who take it suffers blood clots serious enough to require hospitalization. The mortality rate was approximately 1 in 67,000 for women aged 20 to 34 and 1 in 25,000 for women aged 35 to 44.

Nelson said that the package inserts, which the pharmaceutical companies were required to send with their shipments to druggists but which were not at the same time passed on to consumers, warned of "skin blotches, liver damage, mental depression, jaundice, breakthrough bleeding, loss of the sex drive and a very large number of other serious adverse reactions associated with use of the pill." However, Nelson added, "It appears evident that a substantial number of users are not advised of any of the health hazards or side effects." One of the provocations for the hearings, which put me in an odd position, was the publication of my book *The Doctors' Case Against the Pill*, a copy of which was delivered personally to Senator Nelson. At his request, I briefed him and his staff economist, Ben Gordon, privately.

It puzzled me to hear people conclude that Senator Nelson was against the pill when he had, in fact, described it as "effective and convenient," and he never made the slightest suggestion of banning it. However, he did want to give users a chance to make up their own minds, to weigh their personal benefits and risks. It could even be argued that in promoting informed consent, he was taking a stand *for* the pill. That is, if women who knew they were at high risk voluntarily counted themselves out, the pill could have won more trust by those who remained on it. Further, informed women who suffered certain side effects—e.g., dizziness and double vision, possible warnings of a stroke—would know enough to get off the pill and go to an emergency room.

In conducting the hearings, Nelson did not question whether the pill held risks. That fact had already been established, especially in England, where all high-dose brands of the pill had been removed from the Health

Service formulary. Rather, Nelson's purpose was to keep everyone up-to-date. This was, after all, the first time in history that so many healthy young people had been prescribed so powerful a drug for long-term use.

The hearings began on January 14, 1970. As it happened, Senator Bob Dole was in Kansas at the time, but he sent a letter recording his displeasure that Nelson would start without him. In the letter, Dole could not resist reminding Nelson of the "population bomb": "I can safely say that I share with the chairman a deep concern for the national and world problems of overpopulation and environmental health. It is apparent that at the present time the oral contraceptives are important weapons in the struggle to achieve some control over our ability to multiply ourselves into chaos."

Dole also noted that we "must not needlessly frighten millions of women into disregarding the considered judgment of their physicians. . . . Let us show some sympathy for the beleaguered physicians."

The words *needlessly frighten* were repeated over and over by Nelson's critics. I never understood what they meant by *needlessly*. Did they really think that all the studies were wrong, and that no blood clots or strokes were taking place in otherwise healthy young women? Or did they think that women would be scared to death by negative information, even if it was accurate, and that it would be better to die from blood clots than from fright?

Needlessly frighten became a buzz phrase not only during the hearings but also afterward, separating those who valued fairness, evidence, informed consent, and/or women's health rights from those who had other priorities . . . such as population control, pharmaceutical profits, or, if a doctor, maintaining the obedience and blind trust of patients. The battle lines were drawn there in the packed hearing room, but two developments arose that Nelson could not have anticipated. The first was that demonstrations by militant feminists succeeded in bringing a lot of flourish and flavor to the proceedings, turning up the volume on the publicity and in the end securing the patient-information leaflets that Nelson favored but for all his power was unable to bring off. And the second was that some of his loyal friends and colleagues who normally stood with him on drug-industry malfeasance began backing away—in particular, certain of the environmentalists, who, due to the worldwide population explosion, supported "diplomatic immunity" for the pill.

Ironically, it was this population issue raised at the hearings that led to a revelation few Americans had previously been aware of: In its ten years on the market, the pill had failed abysmally in the Third World. Almost all its loyal users were affluent, educated women in the developed countries (the same class of women who opted for the estrogen youth pill). Nelson was long aware that the contraceptive pill was making little dent in world population, for, in the words of *The Washington Post*'s Morton Mintz, he "happens to be one of the most ardent and articulate supporters of family planning on Capitol Hill." Now the senator's careful questions elicited some startling admissions from such well-informed authorities as Dr. Louis Hellman, chairman of the FDA's Advisory Committee on Obstetrics and Gynecology, who testified: "About 18 million people in the world probably use these compounds now. Most of them, as you might imagine, are in the developed countries. The problem in the undeveloped countries [is] they are reluctant to use for a national program products for which we have emphasized certain hazards."

And yet, Phyllis Piotrow, former executive director of the Population Crisis Committee, found it necessary to suggest there would be a crop of "Nelson babies" who, being unwanted, would be beaten by their parents. This provoked reporter Morton Mintz to suggest that, in revenge, admirers of Nelson might wish to personalize disorders caused by the pill as "Piotrow strokes" or "Dole thromboembolisms."

There was a storm of criticism against Gaylord Nelson, but he managed to keep his eye on the main event. He liked to quote a survey taken by *Newsweek* on February 9, 1970, that said two out of every three women on the pill had told poll takers that their doctors had not advised them of the risks. That sort of information reconfirmed the senator's belief that his hearings were worthwhile and necessary. If he made new enemies but saved some women's lives in the process, he would settle for that.

CHAPTER 9

LADIES' NIGHT OUT

They met at an antiwar rally. When Alice Jacobson and Philip Wolfson married in 1968, they hardly had "two nickels to rub together," but they ran up a big bill for furniture at Bloomingdale's because they had faith that a revolution was blowing in the wind.

He was a young doctor in training. She was an activist in several 1960s movements, including ban-the-bomb and civil rights, as well as a member of one of the first women's liberation consciousness-raising groups. A graduate of Barnard and a Fulbright scholar, Alice was both brainy and cute. Their wedding pre-dated the era when women like Alice held on to their maiden names and called themselves "Ms.," but Dr. and Mrs. Wolfson were a quintessential counterculture couple. In 1969, when he was drafted into the Public Health Service, the newlyweds relocated from New York to Washington, D.C. At the time of Senator Nelson's pill hearings, the Wolfsons and their designer chairs and couches shared a large house with eight or ten other people. Philip was the only resident with a steady paycheck. Alice devoted increasing time to her studies of women's liberation. Twenty years later, as if deliberately timed to coincide with her divorce, she made the final payment to Bloomingdale's.

"It's important to explain," Alice reflects today, "what it meant to be a young radical living in Washington in those times. All of us lived fairly inexpensive marginal lives, living in communes, sharing resources, since none of us worked at full-time jobs. We had political meetings all day long. Whenever we heard about anything that was happening, we would just go up to Capitol Hill to check it out. The week of the pill hearings, the Women's Liberation Health Committee was having a meeting. Discussing whether or not to attend the pill hearings sparked personal conversations about our own experiences with the pill. All four or five of us had taken the pill at one time, but all had discontinued it because we had experienced unpleasant side effects. None of us, luckily, had become severely ill. At that time, we didn't even know you could. My own side effect had been hair loss. I had gone to several doctors about it, concerned that I would be going bald in my twenties. None of the doctors related the hair loss to the pill until I made the connection. The other women in the group had experienced similar problems. We were curious. We went to the Hill to get information. We left having started a social movement."

Alice wasn't exaggerating. At seven o'clock on the evening of January 14, 1970, she and her companions were prominently featured by all three television networks on the evening news. One particular part of their uninvited, unauthorized, spontaneous testimonials—oft repeated, oft recalled, and put on the air that evening by both ABC and CBS— was: "All of the women here have suffered ill effects of the pill. And we were told by the doctors, while suffering these effects, and afterwards, to go on taking the pill."

In the coming weeks, their voices, their statements, their photographs, their commentaries, and their bulletins would be carried again and again by the major media around the world. Six months later, a portrait of Alice appeared on the cover of an AMA leaflet for patients called "What You Should Know About the Pill." Three million copies were printed.

THE BOSTON TEA PARTY OF THE WOMEN'S HEALTH MOVEMENT

DAY 1: ROOM 318, OLD SENATE OFFICE BUILDING, OPENING AT 9:40 A.M.

I first glimpsed Alice from my seat at the press table at the front of the Senate Hearing Room. Dr. Marvin Legator, chief of the Cell Biology Branch at the FDA's Division of Pharmacology, had just completed some alarming testimony on how the pill might be causing genetic damage. Senator Nelson was introducing the next witness, Dr. David Carr, a Canadian professor who'd found a "striking increase in a rare chromosomal defect known as triploidy among the babies of women who conceive within six months of going off the pill. Most of the babies with this defect die in the womb or at birth." Suddenly, as the government record notes: "There was a disturbance from some women in the audience." Someone asked, "Why are there no patients testifying at these hearings?"

I swung around and noticed five young women—including Alice—one of them very pregnant. I would learn that she was Marilyn Webb, founder of *Off Our Backs*, a fledgling newspaper that eventually came to be known as "*The New York Times* of the women's movement."

Alice was the most fiery and persistent, the leader to whom the others looked for cues. These were radical women in their mid-twenties committing civil disobedience, but they didn't look the part. They wore what they called their "straight-lady" clothes. Their hair was clean and shiny. Maybe they even had lipstick on. I'd heard that groups like theirs, women like them, were getting together in cities across the country, from Los Angeles to Boston, to discuss, among other matters, body issues such as birth control, gynecology, and of course the female orgasm. (The Boston group had already begun writing *Our Bodies, Ourselves*, which they would soon self-publish on newsprint.) The key to consciousness-raising on body issues was to speak the unvarnished truth about one's own experiences. Were you faking orgasms? Admit it. Did you get sick on the pill and did your doctor tell you that your symptoms couldn't be from the pill? Don't believe him. Compare notes with your friends.

As a mere uptown feminist—or, to be more accurate, a sympathizer—I was tickled to meet these downtown feminists. (The terminology derives from New York City geography. The Mongol Horde radicals were based in Greenwich Village, the respectable NOW types on the Upper West or East Sides.) I hadn't even joined NOW, believing at the time that journalists should stay clear of political groups. However, I did report enthusiastically on the press conference announcing the launch of NOW that Betty Friedan had held in her apartment at the Dakota on Central Park West.

When I turned to check out the disturbances, so did the rest of the people at the press table, most of them photographers, reporters, and cameramen who quickly shifted their attention from Nelson and his official witness, Dr. Carr, to the Wolfson women committing civil disobedience right there in the Senate, presenting their spontaneous testimony based not on scientific research but on their own life experiences. The women were escorted out by guards, and trailed by more than half the press.

Senator Nelson was nonplussed. He was the most left-leaning senator of his time, perhaps even the most honorable, but he was not quite a man of the people in the manner of Lincoln or Harry Truman or Bobby Kennedy or Bill Clinton. As he'd said to the intruders: "I think you are prejudicing your own case. I might suggest to you ladies that we cannot hear all the viewpoints at once. I imagine there might be ten thousand people who would like to testify. We will have to decide. If you ladies wish to talk to me afterward, please come and see me . . . you girls have a little caucus and decide which will talk one at a time, we can then decide what ladies will testify." He never did invite them to testify; however, he repeatedly invited the drug manufacturers, all of whom declined.

Wolfson told me later that they hadn't planned to interrupt the hearings on that first day; their outburst was utterly spontaneous. But from day one, it was obvious that their disruptions drummed up far more sympathy and publicity than any formal testimony might have. By the time the hearings were over, it was evident that Alice and her coconspirators had unleashed a health activism that was igniting women everywhere. Twenty-five years later, Charles Mann would write in *Science*: "Even as the hearings bared the pill's safety defects, the dissent helped launch a political movement focusing on women's health."

At the start of the disturbance, several men at the press tables had seemed confused as to why the women were upset. One called in to his editor: "These women are rioting because they are terrified that their birth control pills will be taken away." But by evening, once the Wolfson women had held their press conference and submitted to multiple interviews, the group had won the understanding and respect of a surprising number of strait-laced journalists. Even Walter Cronkite had some fun reporting that "almost nine million women in America, and ten million elsewhere, are taking the pill each day, in the words of one expert 'as automatically as chickens eating corn.'"

It was quite a study, seeing how these famous doctors, the witnesses, were so frequently outwitted by the uppity women who kept interrupting them. The women were smart (one of them, Charlotte Bunch, went on to join the Center for Women's Global Leadership, where her efforts through the UN have helped make domestic violence recognized as a crime all over the world). Sometimes as many as thirty would show up: For strategic reasons, it was important to bring in new faces. The women would scatter themselves in the middle of long rows, making it seem more difficult for the guards to reach them and drag them out, thus extending the length of their disruptions.

So successfully did D.C. Women's Liberation make its case that hearings on medical topics that excluded testimony from patients would soon become a thing of the past. But the Boston Tea Party of the women's health movement went far beyond establishing a patient's right to testify before Congress. It led to the opening up of consumer access to information on all prescription drugs, to patient participation on FDA committees, and it helped to determine how to move forward with NIH and other government clinical trials. It also exerted influence on a wide range of other issues—from where money should be spent to how consent forms should be worded. Ultimately, the group succeeded in shifting some power from entrenched interests to ordinary people . . . and patients.

AN ACTIVIST FINDS AN ALLY

It was Day 5, January 23, in Room 2221 of the New Senate Office Building when Nelson took up the mysteries of hormones and metabolism. His first witness, Dr. Hilton Salhanick, had chaired a famous international conference at Harvard in December 1968. In all, fifty-five metabolism researchers presented their findings, and they were grim. It turned out that "no tissue or organ system" is free from some change or effects when a woman takes the pill. As one young Englishman reported afterward, many of the assembled scientists had been inclined to think that the one particular system on which each was personally working might be the only one affected by the pill. "It was a shock to sit there for five days and listen to all those papers. I wasn't the only one who called home long-distance and advised my wife to stop the pill at once."

Then it was Dr. Philip Corfman's turn to testify. The director of the Center for Population Research at NIH as well as a member of the powerful FDA advisory committee that monitored the pill, he described a recent task-force report discussing the pill's effects on the liver, such as causing jaundice; also the common disturbances it causes in sugar metabolism; its effects on thyroid and adrenal gland function; the changes it causes in blood vessels and blood clotting, and in the way the body handles fat, water, salt, and various minerals such as calcium, magnesium, copper, and zinc; and the changes it can bring to bear on lung function and in the central nervous system, including causing depression and headaches. This was shocking information for women in the audience to absorb. Such changes sounded as if they could be very serious over the long run. None of their doctors had mentioned these side effects, if they even knew about them.

As had come to be expected, up jumped the protestors, some thirty of them, one or two at a time, in a measured pattern, and all three networks would feature them yet again on the evening news.

Nelson instructed the guards to clear the room. An AP photo, widely reproduced, captured a guard in what looks like a hand-to-hand struggle with the still very pregnant Marilyn Webb. Nonetheless, Nelson decided to readmit the press, but beyond that, "the public and its virago element were not welcomed back."

Dr. Corfman was fascinated by the protestors and filled with respect for them. And unlike the others who testified—who frowned or pretended not to notice or, once in a while, mumbled something unkind—when Nelson calmed himself and told Corfman, "Doctor, go ahead, you may proceed," our government's highest-ranked population expert responded, with perhaps a touch of reproach toward Nelson, "Incidentally, some of the questions placed by the people who interrupted our hearing were quite important."

To succeed in its long-term goals, any social movement must have a respectable branch and a more radical one. The moderate feminists got nowhere much until the downtown feminists caused trouble, which made the demands of the uptowners appear to be reasonable. Another necessity is a loyal friend on the inside, a true believer in the cause, an ally.

Phillip Corfman was such a person. He had married his college sweetheart, Eunice Luccock, a feminist. His mother and his grandmother were feminists too. His family was long associated with Oberlin, America's first coed college and a spawning ground for nineteenth-century suffragists such as Lucy Stone. It was natural for Corfman to agree with many of Alice Wolfson's goals. He and Eunice would smooth the way for the women's health movement at every opportunity. Eventually, as you will see, he would perform a little sleight-of-hand for the good of the hormonal experiment known as the Women's Health Initiative Trial.

CHAPTER 10

IF THE TRUTH BE TOLD

In The New York Times, *Dr. Howard A. Rusk described the hearings* as "an epidemic of anxiety that has spread like wildfire, robbing women of their peace of mind." Many establishment doctors testified, but one of them, however unintentionally, did the most to convince women that they were being deceived.

He was Dr. Robert Kistner.

DR. KISTNER AND THE SILENCE THAT COULD KILL YOU

One of the hearing's most defining moments, dramatically raising both consciousness and eyebrows, was the Day 2 testimony of Dr. Robert Kistner, a Harvard professor, a witness for the drug industry in pill cases, and the author of a popular book, *The Pill: Fact or Fallacy?*

Kistner had mentioned that he never tried to whitewash minor side effects of the pill and often gave patients medication to correct them. After his formal testimony, Kistner was questioned by Senator Thomas McIntyre of New Hampshire.

Senator Thomas McIntyre:

Dr. Kistner, in your own practice do you regularly inform a woman of potential side effects before starting her on the pill?

Dr. Robert Kistner:

Yes . . . I tell her about the side effects . . . weight gain . . . edema and I may even give a prescription for this . . . but I wouldn't go through the list of possible complications. . . . I don't believe it is good medical practice. . . . I wouldn't say, "Now, you may die of blood clotting or you may get hepatitis."

Senator McIntyre:

Well, Doctor, there is one thing that occurs to me, could you distinguish for me the difference between a side effect and a complication?

Dr. Kistner:

Yes. A side effect of a drug is one that is generally accepted as occurring in some individuals as an undesirable effect other than that for which the drug is given. If one takes estrogen, one frequently becomes nauseated. Estrogen "pulls in" sodium and some women don't excrete the excess fluid and they become edematous and "blow up." These are side effects. But if a woman takes estrogen and gets a blood clot and dies, that is a complication.

Senator McIntyre:

That is more than a complication.

TURNING POINT

Kistner was well liked and well respected, a popular professor with a caring manner, and he was one of the first, as a colleague of John Rock at Harvard, to do research on the pill back in the mid-1950s. And to the shock of everyone in the jam-packed hearing room, he had just confirmed the litany of wrongs the Wolfson women had complained about the day before—the secrecy, the patronization, the evasiveness that placed women in harm's way.

Senator McIntyre's questions and Dr. Kistner's answers marked the defining moment that won the public over to a belief in informed consent. To be sure, the demand for it reached such a pitch that on March 4, 1970, the ninth and final day of the hearing, FDA Commissioner Dr. Charles Edwards declared, "I have come to the conclusion that the information being supplied to the patient in the case of the oral contraceptive is insufficient, and that a reevaluation of our present policies is in order. . . . I have with me today . . . a leaflet designed to reinforce the information provided to the patient by her physician."

This excellent document of 600 words was entitled "What You Should Know About Birth Control Pills."

WHAT YOU SHOULD KNOW ABOUT BIRTH CONTROL PILLS
(ORAL CONTRACEPTIVE PRODUCTS)
All of the oral contraceptive pills are highly effective for preventing pregnancy when taken according to the approved

directions. Your doctor has taken your medical history and has given you a careful physical examination. He has discussed with you the risks of oral contraceptives and has decided that you can take this drug safely.

This leaflet is your reminder of what your doctor has told you. Keep it handy and talk to him if you think you are experiencing any of the conditions you find described.

A Warning About Blood Clots

There is a definite association between blood-clotting disorders and the use of oral contraceptives. The risk of this complication is six times higher for users than for nonusers. The majority of blood-clotting disorders are not fatal. The estimated death rate from blood clotting in women *not* taking the pill is 1 in 200,000 each year; for users, the death rate is about 6 in 200,000. Women who have or who have had blood clots in the legs, lung, or brain should not take this drug. You should stop taking it and call your doctor immediately if you develop severe leg or chest pain, if you cough up blood, if you experience sudden and severe headaches, or if you cannot see clearly.

Who Should Not Take Birth Control Pills

Besides women who have or who have had blood clots, women who should not use oral contraceptives are those who have serious liver disease, cancer of the breast or certain other cancers, and vaginal bleeding of unknown cause.

Special Problems

If you have heart or kidney disease, asthma, high blood pressure, diabetes, epilepsy, fibroids of the uterus, migraine headaches, or if you have had any problems with mental depression, your doctor has indicated you need special supervision while taking oral contraceptives. Even if you don't have special problems, he will want to see you regularly to check your blood pressure, examine your breasts, and make certain other tests.

When you take the pill as directed, you should have your period each month. If you miss a period, and if you are sure you have been taking the pill as directed, continue your schedule. If you have not been taking the pill as directed and if you miss one period, stop taking it and call your doctor. If you miss two periods, see your doctor even though you have been taking the pill as directed. When you stop taking the pill, your periods may be irregular for some time. During this time, you may have trouble becoming pregnant.

If you have had a baby, whom you are breastfeeding, you should know that if you start taking the pill its hormones are in your milk. The pill may also cause a decrease in your milk flow. After you have had a baby, check with your doctor before starting to take oral contraceptives again.

What to Expect

Oral contraceptives normally produce certain reactions that are more frequent the first few weeks after you start taking them. You may notice unexpected bleeding or spotting and experience changes in your period. Your breasts may feel tender, look larger, and discharge slightly. Some women gain weight while others lose it. You may also have episodes of nausea and vomiting. You may notice a darkening of the skin in certain areas.

Other Reactions to Oral Contraceptives

In addition to blood clots, other reactions produced by the pill may be serious. These include mental depression, swelling, skin rash, jaundice or yellow pigment in your eyes, an increase in blood pressure, and an increase in the sugar content of your blood similar to that seen in diabetes.

Possible Reactions

Women taking the pill have reported headaches, nervousness, dizziness, fatigue, and backache. Changes in appetite and sex drive, pain when urinating, growth of more body hair, loss of scalp hair, and nervousness and irritability before the period also have been reported. These reactions may or may not be directly related to the pill.

Note About Cancer

Scientists know the hormones in the pill (estrogen and progesterone) have caused cancer in animals, but they have no

> proof that the pill causes cancer in humans. Because your doc-
> tor knows this, he will want to examine you regularly.

The full text was published in *The New York Times* and many other papers. The wording was helpful and clear, and the document was greeted with enormous gratitude by the pill-using public. Yet within weeks, it was derailed, in a scandalous manner, by that unholy trio of organized medi-cine, drug manufacturers, and extremist population controllers.

Alice Wolfson, with daring assistance from two members of the FDA's Advisory Committee—Dr. Roy Hertz and Dr. Philip Corfman—as well as help from sympathetic reporters at *The Washington Post* and *Star*, and even (after another sit-in) HEW Secretary Robert Finch, would swing back into action and save the warning, though in a much abbreviated and harder to read form.

CHAPTER 11

ALICE KEEPS BUSY AND THE FDA COMES THROUGH

Dr. Edwards has said he abandoned "What You Should Know . . ." because it contains "too much clinical material" and because "it wasn't our job to play doctor or to scare people away from the Pill." He denied he was pressured by top HEW officials.

—*THE WASHINGTON POST*, April 6, 1970

Flyers advertising the Women's Hearings on the pill (held at a church in Washington three days after the Senate hearings ended on March 4) read: "The Pill: Is it a menace, a no-no, or a girl's best friend?" The promotions further explained, "We are not opposed to oral contraception for men or for women. We are opposed to unsafe contraceptives foisted on uninformed women for the profit of the drug and medical industries, and for the convenience of men." Of course the flyers also announced, as was de rigueur in those days at feminist events, that "free child care will be available." Thanks to Commissioner Edwards's initial bold move, the audience and the speakers felt quite empowered. They looked forward to a new era where women—in fact, all patients—would be partners in their own health care.

But the jubilation was brief. FDA Commissioner Edwards had told the Senate subcommittee that his 600-word document would be placed within ten days in the *Federal Register* "so all interested parties will have an opportunity to comment on it." However, on March 24, the press reported that Edwards had reneged. Senator Thomas McIntyre, who had so adroitly questioned Dr. Kistner, sent an official protest:

> As a member of the subcommittee I had been concerned that women who might be considering use of the Pill were not being provided the necessary information concerning its known and potential dangers to enable them to make an informed and rational decision as to whether they wanted to use the pill or some other method of contraception. I thought that the labeling proposed by Commissioner Edwards at the hearings went a long way toward answering this need. I anticipated that it would be published in essentially the same form in the *Federal Register* so that all interested parties would have opportunity to comment before the order was finalized."
>
> Needless to say, I was amazed to hear that the agency had shortened the label statement from 600 words to 90 words, and deleted much of the essential information even before the order was published.

What could have gone wrong? According to *The New York Times*, "Dr. Edwards ruffled bureaucratic feathers when he told the Senate subcommittee about the leaflet and its specific warning without first informing his superior, Dr. Roger Egeberg, Assistant Secretary of Health, Education and Welfare (now a department of HSS)." Then Gerald Dorman, president of the American Medical Association, "complained to Dr. Egeberg and HEW Secretary Finch that the leaflet would interfere with the doctor-patient relationship and possibly could lead to malpractice suits."

When queried on this point by Stuart Auerbach of *The Washington Post*, Frank Acosta, the FDA's press spokesman, stated, "Dr. Egeberg thought it was too long." Auerbach also uncovered protests from drug companies, "who thought the warning gave too much emphasis to the dangers of the pill, and not enough to its benefits." The third shoe, Auerbach found, was dropped by "agencies such as Planned Parenthood, concerned about the world population explosion and fearful that the pill warning would lead to unwanted pregnancies." In the end, Auerbach reached the conclusion that it was the AMA, above all, that succeeded in derailing the 600-word version of "What You Should Know About Birth Control Pills."

In their strange and strained alliance, Gaylord Nelson and Alice Wolfson—he representing the power of the U.S. Senate, she the growing demands of women's lib, both of them acting and reacting with extraordinary smarts and speed—had won round one against the conjoint forces of the AMA, the oral-contraceptive manufacturers such as Searle, Syntex, and Ortho, as well as those so devoted to population control that they upheld the "diplomatic immunity" of the pill.

The Wolfson women's first protest following the withdrawal of "What You Should Know" took place on April 1, 1970. It was reported by Morton Mintz in *The Washington Post* on April 6:

An entirely new warning to users of the Pill has been recommended to the Food and Drug Administration by its outside advisors on birth control. . . . The recommended new warning resulted from a hitherto undisclosed development last Wednesday—the invasion by two members of the Women's Liberation Movement of a closed meeting of the Advisory Committee on Obstetrics and Gynecology at FDA headquarters in Rockville. After hearing the Women's Liberation protests, Dr. Roy Hertz, a committee member, wrote this draft for a sticker to be affixed to every package of pills:

"Do not take these pills without your doctor's continued supervision. Contact him if you experience any unusual symptoms, particularly the following: 1. Severe headache. 2. Blurred vision. 3. Pain in the legs. 4. Pain in the chest or cough. 5. Irregular or missed periods."

THE STORY BEHIND THE STICKER

The sticker—even shorter than the abbreviated version of "What You Should Know" but more concise and more easily read—was perhaps the first victory in the political war that Dr. Corfman, a white knight of sorts, would fight to perfection. Dr. Roy Hertz, Corfman's friend and colleague on the FDA advisory committee and a world authority on hormonal cancers, shared the belief that pill users had every right to know the worst that could befall them. Understanding the powers marshaled against full disclosure, they concluded that something very short and pertinent had the best chance of making the cut. They composed the new mini-warning and found a strategy to float it. Corfman called me in New York, mentioning the time and place the committee would hold a meeting to discuss the future of "What You Should Know About Birth Control Pills." He figured, correctly, that I would tell Alice and that she might feel compelled to drop by, which of course she did. While she was there, Hertz made his dramatic announcement, counting on Alice to leak it to Morton Mintz. But it was one thing for Hertz and Corfman to devise such a worthy compromise and make it known. Now there must be more heat.

Alice's next stop was the office of President Nixon's secretary of HEW, Robert Finch, who had a liberal reputation. "We had watched and waited," said Alice, "but when nothing appeared in the *Federal Register*, we held a sit-in at the office of Secretary Finch. We sat around, those of us with babies publicly nursing in the rather posh waiting room, and refused to move until he agreed to schedule a meeting with us. I remember several employees walking in, taking one look at us, and one of them said, 'Oh, Lordy, the revolution has come to HEW.'"

On April 8, the FDA finally published a version of "What You Should Know" in the *Federal Register*. It was the third draft, and back up to 120 words, including Dr. Hertz's brief, five-point lifesaving attention-grabber to be affixed right on the packet. Over 800 letters were received, addressed to Finch, to Edwards, and to the Hearing Clerk in Rockville, Maryland. More than half protested the abridgment of the proposed text. In fact, on April 27, Secretary Finch sent me a letter stating that my book had influenced him to "strengthen the language in the final warning. . . . I recognize that you and your associates feel that this is still inadequate," he said, "but I hope you will agree that it is an improvement over the second draft."

I did agree; this version had teeth. Soon after, Finch was removed as HEW secretary and transferred to the White House as a presidential advisor. Dr. Herbert Ley, former FDA commissioner, also lost his job, after he endorsed my book, and Nelson got himself caught in a backlash that almost threatened the success of his lifelong dream for an Earth Day. I wondered if *The Doctors' Case Against the Pill* should have carried a warning: "This book may be dangerous to your career."

The final warning, a minimal package insert, was a disappointment to many, but thanks to the Hertz/Corfman/Wolfson caper—and the last-minute support of Finch—the critical and lifesaving message was pasted to the outside of the packet, with an insert inside calling attention to the longer version by informing patients that further information was available. Deaths from the pill began to fall at once, yet doctors still saw the warning as a serious encroachment. It represented "an important turning point in the doctor-patient relationship," according to Elizabeth Siegel Watkins. "Patients had demanded the right to know about the medications prescribed for them, and the package insert legitimized this claim." In addition, an 800-word booklet jointly written by the AMA, FDA, and ACOG, and much like Commissioner Edwards's original, was distributed to doctors to give to their patients if they wished. The woman on the cover of the booklet looked exactly like Alice.

I thought the booklet was quite good and spent a lot of time button-holing women to find out if they had received it. Those who went to clinics often did; those who went to private doctors usually did not. However, by the late 1970s, consumers did get a longer and more comprehensive document dispensed by pharmacists. Unfortunately, it was more legalistic, more technical, and altogether less user-friendly than Dr. Edwards's original 1970 "What You Should Know."

TAKING HORMONES AND WOMEN'S HEALTH

On December 16, 1975, Alice Wolfson and I, with three other women— Belita Cowan, Dr. Mary Howell, and Dr. Phyllis Chesler—founded a Washington-based organization we called the National Women's Health Network. We included in our charter that under no circumstances would we accept drug-company money, and gathered on the front steps of the FDA in Rockville, Maryland, to hold a memorial service for all the women who'd died from unnecessary estrogen products in the Greatest Experiment. Theologians, including Mary Daly, made introductions. The first mourner was twenty-one-year-old Sherry L., a DES daughter, exposed to the hormone in her mother's womb, who consequently developed cervical abnormalities and a possibly precancerous condition. Like 1.5 million other DES daughters in the United States, she lived in fear and in mourning for those who had died from the rare cancer that derives from prenatal exposure. Nor was Premarin forgotten. I contributed a few words about Sally. Jim Luggen, a young widower from Dayton, Ohio, held up a photo of his beautiful wife, Dona Jean Walter, who had died from a pulmonary embolism that her doctors attributed to the pill. Dr. Richard Crout, the head of the FDA Bureau of Drugs, had come out to listen. I thought I saw tears in his eyes when Luggen was speaking.

As the ceremony ended, Crout promised that he would get us mandated warnings on all estrogen products, and he did. He had introduced himself to me as an Oberlin alumnus and a friend of Phil and Eunice Corfman, the latter a founding member of the National Women's Health Network. When she died in 1980, her family and friends endowed an internship in her name.

The National Women's Health Network established an information clearinghouse. The staff and the board closely monitored menopause estrogens and put out a regular publication called *Taking Hormones and Women's Health*. When, in June 1990, Wyeth-Ayerst asked the FDA to approve the use of Premarin in women to prevent heart disease without evidence from randomized controlled trials to support this indication, no professional society opposed the request, but the NWHN spoke against it.

Cindy Pearson, then the program director, was the most vigorous dissenter. She charged Wyeth with sexism, pointing out that no drug had ever been approved for this purpose in men without a quality clinical trial. The FDA advisory committee voted to approve the Wyeth request. Commenting on the data, committee chairman Dr. Barbara Hulka, of the University of North Carolina School of Public Health, said, "From the standpoint of epidemiology and the many impressive analytic studies that have been done, the findings are impressive."

Philip Corfman had by now moved from NIH to the FDA and was a member of the staff handling the proposal. He was also the liaison with the advisory committee and secretary at the meetings. He and other members of the staff, including Drs. Solomon Sobel and Linda Golden, agreed with Pearson that the observational studies lacked conviction, and Corfman asked the advisory committee if they wished to recommend a large clinical trial. They agreed, not thinking of this as a prerequisite to the labeling upgrade sought by Wyeth-Ayerst.

But the staff put a different interpretation on the move. They took the call for clinical trials as a caution to wait for clearer results. Having exercised a pocket veto, they didn't put the upgrade through. Nearly a year passed, to the displeasure of Wyeth and some members of the advisory committee. The situation came to a head in April at a hearing of a Senate subcommittee on aging, where the FDA was called on to defend its lack of action on Premarin as a heart-problem deterrent. Dr. Bruce Burlington, deputy director of the FDA Office of Drug Evaluation, described by a former colleague as having a "very sharp and keen mind," testified that "the studies that are available on Premarin's cardiovascular effects do not constitute randomized prospective clinical trials that offer hard data. . . . The epidemiologic studies and cohort studies have statistical and methodological faults that make interpretations difficult." Burlington said that he applauded an initiative recently announced by the NIH to look prospectively at the long-term effects of hormone therapy on cardiovascular disease as well as osteoporosis, breast cancer, and stroke. Dr. Solomon Sobel accompanied Burlington to the hearing and also emphasized that a "large prospective randomized study will do a great deal to help us define that issue."

And so it was that a tiny band of dedicated, underpaid FDA scientists, reluctant to approve an indication in which they did not believe, and given the opportunity by Pearson to take the evidence of a double standard and run with it, made the unusual move of tabling a near-unanimous recommendation of its advisory committee. The FDA *never approved* the cardioprotective indication of Premarin, and their eloquent statements on the reasons for their reluctance—the same that led Wyeth to supply medication free of charge (a move that failed to pay off)—encouraged Congress to fund the hugely expensive Women's Health Initiative.

What has happened to the people involved? Cindy Pearson, the program director of the National Women's Health Network when she helped to block the cardioprotective approval, is now the organization's tremendously well-respected executive director. Dr. Solomon Sobel is still at the FDA. Dr. Phil Corfman retired but is still in constant demand as a consultant on international family-planning programs. As for Dr. Bruce Burlington, he was promoted to director of the FDA's Center for Devices and Radiological Health, where he did an outstanding job of straightening out a division that had been in chaos, but eventually was passed over for commissioner. In the interim, he resorted to moonlighting at a hospital emergency room. "Bruce's moonlighting was very uncommon," according to a colleague at the FDA. "But he had alimony to pay and five kids to support. He needed the cash."

On March 15, 1999, Wyeth-Ayerst issued this press release:

Wyeth-Ayerst Laboratories, the pharmaceutical division of American Home Products Corporation (NYSE: AHP), announced today that Bruce Burlington, M.D., has joined the Company as Senior Vice President, Global Regulatory Affairs for Pharmaceuticals, Vaccines, and Biological Products. Dr. Burlington, who will report to Wyeth-Ayerst Research President L. Patrick Gage, Ph.D., has most recently been Director of the Food and Drug Administration's (FDA) Center for Devices and Radiological Health. . . . Dr. Burlington will oversee programs for registration of products worldwide. Dr. Burlington comes to the Company with 17 years of experience at the FDA.

Wyeth did not mention how many multiples of his FDA salary its former nemesis and new vice president would receive, but (like a virgin bride) those FDA veterans who were extra-tough on industry seem to get the best offers and command the highest prices when they switch.

And what about Alice? She moved to San Francisco in 1977 when her sons were two and five. She remained on the Board of the National Women's Health Network and also became a local health activist in the Bay Area. In 1988, at age sixteen, her older son Noah died of leukemia, after which her marriage failed. She went on to become a lawyer representing patients against insurance companies. And yes, she still gets to the FDA frequently, but she doesn't have to push her way in or hold up placards or speak out of turn anymore. As smart and original as ever, she is the consumer representative on the highly technical Biological Response Modifiers Advisory Committee, which oversees such matters as gene therapy. I'm glad she's there watching out for us.

PART II

WHAT DO WE KNOW NOW?

Introduction II:
Between a Rock and
a Hard Place

I don't think the issue has been concluded at all. The last word has
certainly not been said.

—Virginia Lupkin, M.D., who at age eighty-five gave up Premarin for
three weeks and went back on

There are many similarities between the Pill Panic of 1970 and the
Prempro Panic of 2002, including three outcomes you can count on:

- The drug companies will land on their feet.
- The patients will remain confused and conflicted.
- The "messengers," such as Gaylord Nelson in the Senate
  and Dr. Jacques Rossouw at NIH, will continue to be
  vilified for their good deeds.

In the first part of this book, I described how the Greatest Experiment came about, as I witnessed it. In this part, we will look at what we know now. Much is still tentative, but many important things have been confirmed. Estrogen does *not* prevent heart disease and does increase the risks of hormone-dependent cancers. Many other long-held beliefs are up for grabs. For example, the doctors who claim that estrogen enables a woman to have great sex may be mistaken. Of course it takes care of vaginal dryness, but beyond that, it actually may turn off a woman's sex drive. In an article entitled "Estrogen Replacement May Douse Desire" by Women's E-News correspondent Frances Whittelsey, Natallie DeVane, a spokeswoman for Wyeth, stated that both estrogen and progestin may suppress a woman's libido. This reaction is described in the *Physicians' Desk Reference* as simply "changes in libido."

What we all need to do now, patients as well as doctors, is to learn how to evaluate the *quality* of information. The National Institutes of Health has developed a scorecard of what they call evidence, rated A, B, C, and D, which I will explain shortly so that you might utilize it in making your decisions.

For some women, these decisions are very difficult. They feel "in the pink" on estrogen and anywhere from so-so to dreadful without it. I have been interviewing and receiving letters from estrogen users who stopped taking the drug in the summer of 2002 on hearing the news that it may cause more problems than it corrects or prevents. Nobody knows why some two-thirds of former users are doing well without their hormone supplements while others feel a great decline and a great loss. The highest priority, therefore, should be given to research that identifies those who may still need hormones to maintain a good quality of life and those for whom they are irrelevant.

Dr. Virginia Lupkin, still an active and creative medical researcher in her eighties, was on Premarin, progestin, and synthroid for forty years. When she gave up the sex hormones, she had "a negative spike in the direction of increased bone discomfort."

Janet Feldman, also in her eighties and also a user "forever," as she puts it, has long been active in nongovernmental organizations at the United Nations headquarters in New York. She went off hormones but will probably go back on them because "suddenly, I'm now an old lady. I don't swim anymore. I don't go to the UN."

But it isn't only the ultra long-term users who may find themselves out of the pink if they abruptly quit. It can happen to younger women as well. Lori S., a reader of my column in a magazine, wrote to me:

November 12: At age sixty plus, I'm back to hot flashes, my hair is falling out, and my wrinkles are getting wrinkles. Prempro kept me sane and "well preserved" for almost fifteen years. Now I feel that I've aged overnight. November 13: I went "cold turkey." I didn't think it would have mattered in the long run, sort of like giving up smoking. I am tempted to resume but . . . is it worth trading present well-being for possible risks of major health problems down the line? Seems like a no-win situation. Any suggestions?

Yes, I have a suggestion. Doctors must pay attention to the reasons that some women do feel in the pink on hormones. They must listen to their patients and the patients must demand respectful attention from their doctors. And then I hope they will do the research, scientists and volunteers together carrying out high-quality clinical trials to figure out what may underlie the quality-of-life benefits for certain women but by no means all.

Another suggestion. Lori S. might have made a better adjustment if she had tapered off. There are reports that patients who wean themselves

slowly—over two, three months or a full year—have an easier time. Dr.
Bruce Ettinger at Kaiser Permanente in Oakland, California, and Dr.
Charles Debrovner in New York City are collecting data on tapering even
as I write.

On December 12, I received another note from Lori S.:

> I don't want to suffer anymore; I'm going back on. Hopefully one
> day the scientists will be able to separate the harmful properties of
> the drug from the beneficial elements. Until then, I feel as if I'm
> eating a poisoned apple.

Poisoned apple? Perhaps so. In 1995, Dr. Jan-Ake Gustafsson of the
Karolinska Institute in Stockholm discovered that drug companies had
been flying blind, assuming there was only one type of estrogen receptor
(ER) in the female body. Dr. Gustafsson found a second (ER beta) and, as
Dr. Jill Siegfried of the University of Pittsburgh explains, "ER beta is made
from a different gene than ER alpha. ER beta is high in the ovary, the
uterus and in the brain. It is also high in the lung. It is low in the breast."
Further estrogen receptors are being described, including one called
ER-X from Dr. Dominique Toran-Allerand at Columbia Medical School.

What does all this mean for women who take hormones? As an NIH
publication stated in 2002, "Pharmaceutical ambitions to develop new
and better targeted hormone therapies were much hampered by the static
dogma of one single receptor. There were many contradictory effects of
estrogens that seemed difficult to explain. The sudden and unexpected
appearance of ERB on the scene caused somewhat of a catharsis in the
field and offered explanations for old enigmas and controversies." And so,
as Lori S. hopes, safer hormone products may be on the way, but they're
not here yet. There is still more basic research to do.

In January 2003, Dr. Lisa Rarick of the FDA explained the new regulations on estrogen to reporters. It was refreshing that she did not conclude her statement with the old saw "Ask your doctor." To the contrary, Rarick advised taking estrogen for the shortest time possible and then declared that "the individual woman is advised to consider her own situation." Let's not overlook the fact that the doctors failed us by allowing some manufacturers to pull the wool over their eyes. But women, in the end, must make our own decisions. What, then, do we need to know to do so? Mainly, we must learn to tell the good studies from the bad, which is not so difficult once we grasp the basics, beginning with these evidence categories as described by the NIH in terms of Grades A, B, C, and D:

A stands for a "rich body of data" with a consistent pattern of findings from randomized controlled trials. A full-blown A grade requires "substantial number of studies involving substantial number of participants."

B indicates a "limited body of data" from randomized controlled trials. In general, category B pertains when few randomized trials exist, when they are small in size, and when the results are somewhat inconsistent or the population is not identical to the target population to which the recommendations are being made. Such an example would be to make the assumption that women who retain their ovaries benefit as much from estrogen as women who've had their ovaries removed.

C pertains to nonrandomized trials and/or observational studies. If you don't randomize, but merely observe, you will likely find that women on estrogen are less prone to heart disease than those who aren't. Yet as we now know, it was a mistake to attribute this fact to hormones, because women who take estrogen are healthier and more educated to start with, eat more prudently, exercise more, and are less likely to smoke. So be wary of giving too much weight to simple observation.

D refers to expert judgment. This category is used "only in cases where the provision of some guidance is deemed valuable" but where actual studies are nonexistent or weak. For example, it takes for granted that estrogen would help control urinary stress incontinence, because doctors assumed the hormone kept a woman youthful "down there." But clinical trials now indicate that, as with heart disease, the estrogen makes stress incontinence a little bit *more* likely. Yet again, the experts were proved wrong.

How, then, can you learn to distinguish the wrongs from the rights? An excellent way is to turn to the medical literature, the sort that is up-to-date and doesn't talk down to the reader. One such publication is the NIH's 300-page *Women's Health and Menopause: A Comprehensive Report*, available on the website of the National Health Lung and Blood Institute (http//nhlbi.nih.gov/prof/heart/other.menopaus). It is designed for professionals, but with a medical dictionary in hand, you may be able to understand all but the most technical sections. And to my mind, it is *the* place to start giving yourself a free and thorough education.

Getting to the Heart of the Matter: Estrogen, Heart Disease, and the Triumph of Suggestion over Science

Science in the modern world has many uses; its chief use, however, is to provide long words to cover the errors of the rich.

—G. K. Chesterton

The children's game Jenga is a simple but tricky one. To win, competitors must gradually remove one piece at a time from a tower of wooden blocks without causing the tower's collapse. Usually it takes a long time for the blocks to fall and involves eroding the tower until its collapse is inevitable. Sometimes, however, a player will remove a seemingly noncrucial piece early in the game, which will, to the surprise of all the players, bring the whole thing crashing down. When the NIH Women's Health Initiative reported that its participants had experienced a rise in heart disease while taking estrogen, I knew that such a piece had been pulled from the poorly constructed tower of positive hormone therapy evidence.

The medical establishment was incredulous. It shouldn't have been, since, as we've seen, Premarin has never had FDA approval as a heart drug. Never mind that doctors and scientists continued to advocate and prescribe estrogen for both the prevention and treatment of cardiac disease. Despite any solid evidence on the subject, it became perceived knowledge that estrogen was cardioprotective (an assumption that would be rated C under today's NIH categories of evidence). The rationale for the belief was simple: Women who take estrogen live longer than women who do not. Many doctors reasoned that this was likely the work of estrogen.

> The Network strongly opposes the proposed indication for Premarin as a coronary heart disease preventative. Premarin has not been adequately studied and its use for such a purpose would be premature. . . . We believe that Wyeth-Ayerst should be held to the same standard that manufacturers of heart disease medication for men have been held to. A controlled, double-blind clinical trial of appropriate duration and adequate size should be required. When aspirin was being considered a preventative of coronary heart disease in men, 20,000 men were involved in a placebo-controlled trial. Don't we deserve as much?

Harvard Women's Health Watch stated empirically that "estrogen is considered to be responsible for [women's] 15- to 20-year advantage over men in evading coronary artery disease. Not only do most women have little evidence of heart problems during their reproductive years, when estrogen levels are high, but those who take estrogen after menopause seem to have lower rates of heart attack."

During the years between the FDA rejection of Premarin as a heart drug and the negative discoveries about estrogen in the Women's Health Initiative, monthly health newsletters nonetheless played an important role in assuring women of estrogen's cardioprotective value. These newsletters, and other print and Internet sources that summarize recent health findings, have an interesting place as mediator between a potentially complicated medical study and the average reader. They speak colloquially, simply, and confidentially, clearly trying to communicate that they will impart to the reader the straight story on a given issue. This is a dangerous assumption, because many of these publications are directly or indirectly sponsored by industry and can be used as platforms to slant a story or give a particular spin on an issue. Even the many publications that are not industry sponsored and are well intentioned are often guilty at the very least of oversimplification, providing the reader with one opinion of what a study shows without also providing essential contextual information, such as what kind of study it was, how large it was, and how long it lasted.

In the case of estrogen and heart disease, a look at several major health newsletters between 1995 and 2000 provides a valuable lesson in the importance of reading closely and paying particular attention to the words an author chooses to describe a given finding.

The *Harvard Women's Health Watch* article quoted above begins by stating that "by now" a reader is "probably well aware" that estrogen is considered to be responsible for women's comparatively longer average life span. By choosing to start the story this way it is likely that the writer wants the reader to assume that this theory is somehow common and accepted knowledge. While the article goes on to admit that evidence for estrogen's heart-sparing effects is "mostly circumstantial" and "derived, for the most part, from observational studies" rather than from long-term clinical trials, it proceeds to list different ways in which estrogen seems to help the heart, including so-called evidence that estrogen helps raise HDL ("good") cholesterol levels and perhaps increases the body's ability to dissolve blood clots. This last suggestion is particularly troubling because estrogen, like birth control pills, has long been known to increase blood clotting, *not* decrease it.

Another 1995 article, this one in the *University of California at Berkeley Wellness Letter*, uses even stronger language, stating: "It has long been known that estrogen therapy lowers the risk of heart disease after menopause," and it gives no indication that the statement is anything other than documented medical truth.

Newsletters also kept the heart-disease myth alive by focusing on less-sweeping, less-general conclusions, such as the results of numerous small studies that compared the effectiveness of estrogen-only pills on the heart with estrogen/progestin combination pills. Here again, the absence of any significant findings is not made clear. The *University of Texas Lifetime Health Letter*, for one, begins a March 1995 item called "Estrogen-Progestin Combo Benefits the Heart" by stating: "Numerous studies have suggested that post-menopausal estrogen replacement therapy can reduce a woman's risk of heart disease." The use of the word *suggested* is particularly revealing. The article proceeds to give women the "good news" that estrogen/progestin combination pills have been found to have "beneficial effects on heart disease risk factors" equal to those found in estrogen-only pills. The report is interesting because, in comparing the different estrogens, it implies that estrogen is effective for heart disease without providing any initial evidence for either. It also admits that the benefit of estrogen for the heart is only "suggested" but then goes on to assure the reader that one form of estrogen is just as effective as another.

A May 1997 *Consumer Reports on Health* article called "Heart Disease in Women: Special Symptoms, Special Risks" again tells readers that "taking female hormones sharply reduces the risk of coronary disease," adding that "it also eases menopausal symptoms, slashes the risk of osteoporosis, and may decrease the chance of colon cancer, tooth loss, and possibly osteo-arthritis and Alzheimer's disease." In this litany of benefits, only the easing of menopausal symptoms and the prevention of osteoporosis have the distinction of having been FDA-approved uses for the drugs. Disturbingly, the article goes on to say that "for most women, those benefits clearly outweigh the treatment's main drawbacks—renewed menstrual bleeding with some regimens, and possibly a slight increase in the risk of breast cancer and blood clots in the legs and lungs." This analysis raises a major red flag in saying that the benefits outweigh the risks, especially in the unproven off-label reasons to prescribe estrogen. For example, regardless of the effect estrogen seems to have relative to cholesterol, it appears logically inconsistent that something known to cause blood clotting would lower the incidence of heart attack.

THE PRESS: ITS POWER AND PREJUDICES

It is not only newsletters but also newspapers that muddy the coverage of estrogen. I noted in a 1997 article called "The Media and the Menopause Industry" that the September 12, 1991, edition of *The New York Times* gave front page coverage to hopeful news about estrogen and the heart from the Harvard Nurses Health Study. On the other hand, more ominous news on the same subject from the same source was relegated much farther back in the same issue, page 18 (placement is all when it comes to editorializing about the importance of a given finding). Other significant negatives from the Harvard Nurses Health Study—for example, that the risk of asthma doubles in long-term estrogen users—did not make the paper at all. Nor did the *Times*, the paper of record, include reports in October of 1996 that women on lower-dose estrogen continued to face an increased risk of blood clots in the legs and lungs.

The press, whether intentionally fueled by drug-dollar deceit or simply from negligence and oversight, continued for years to report as virtual fact a connection between heart and hormone that did not carry enough weight to justify adding cardiac care to the FDA-approved uses for the drug. This failure of the press to give equal time to the entire spectrum of positions on various hormone issues, including estrogen therapy and heart disease, whether inadvertent or not, nonetheless misled the public. Women, therefore, have good reason to be skeptical of the shock claimed by the medical community when the Women's Health Initiative disproved the ability of estrogen to help the heart. Though insiders had known how limited the evidence was, the positive heart-hormone connection was still presented as a given, which meant that either these doctors and scientists had demonstrated a serious lack of judgment in prescribing estrogen for cardiac purposes or women were not being given the truth.

The first serious blow to the perceived wisdom about estrogen and the heart was reported in the August 19, 1998, issue of the *Journal of the American Medical Association*. The article was based on the Heart and Estrogen/Progestin Replacement Study (HERS), which found that in a group of 2,763 women who had experienced a heart attack, those who were on estrogen suffered more deaths and additional heart attacks in the first two years than those who were not.

Still, many members of the medical community were quick to point out that the findings applied only to women who had already experienced a heart attack, and that in cases where subsequent ones occurred it was only in the first years following the initial episode. As Dr. Diana Petitti wrote in an accompanying editorial, "Physicians need to carefully review the HERS findings, but no woman, including those with coronary heart disease, should abruptly cease use of ERT or HRT because of the HERS results." Health newsletters, too, were generally quick to emphasize the limitations of the study. *Consumer Reports on Health* went so far as to state that "the study did turn up one genuinely significant positive finding that agreed with earlier evidence: hormone therapy produced a sizable rise in 'good' HDL cholesterol levels and a comparable decline in 'bad' LDL cholesterol." To me, that is akin to saying, "The operation was a success, but the patient died."

The *Women's Health Advisor*, a consistently estrogen-friendly publication, carried an article dubbing the HERS findings "puzzling" and insisting that "in fact, data show that HRT can lower the risk of heart attack by as much as 40% and the risk of stroke by as much as 20%." The article went on to assert that "the HERS findings apply only to women who already have heart disease. For the rest of us, estrogen's protective effect is well documented."

Suddenly, however, in April 2000, when the Women's Health Initiative informed the 27,000 women participating in its ongoing hormone-therapy trial that those taking estrogen were at greater risk for heart attack, the language about estrogen vis-à-vis heart disease became much more cautious. Publications such as *The New England Journal of Medicine's Health News* advised readers, "Previous research had suggested that HRT might protect postmenopausal women against heart disease, but the picture has become more complicated in recent years." Yet even then, the *Women's Health Advisor* stopped short of being out and out negative, reminding readers to "bear in mind that the WHI findings are preliminary. It is still too early to rule out the possibility that estrogen can help prevent heart disease."

In 2002, *Women's Health and Menopause: A Comprehensive Approach*, by Drs. Peter Coolins, Nanette K. Wenger, Jacques Rossouw, and Rodolfo Paoletti, was published and stands now as the most reliable assessment of estrogen and risk of heart disease. The publication says that although hormone therapy has been associated with a lower risk of cardio-vascular disease in epidemiological studies, it has not been borne out in clinical trials. The authors also reiterate the seemingly obvious point that given this new information, women should look at lifestyle factors—including the cessation of smoking, increasing physical activity, exercising, improving nutrition, losing and maintaining weight, lowering stress levels, and managing high blood pressure and diabetes—as ways of preventing heart disease. They also recommend alternative pharmacological interven-tion, including beta-blockers, aspirin, statins, and ACE inhibitors, which, they write, "can reduce the risk of cardiovascular events in women." How-ever, these drugs are being questioned as well.

Perhaps one of the most important points the authors make is that "the main causes, prevention, and treatment of CVD [cardiovascular dis-ease] in women are similar to those in men." This conclusion further highlights the issue of gender in the estrogen debacle. However, therapy had always been about treating the natural process of menopause in women as if it were a disease. But now, the doctors conclude, it is better to treat the heart disease specifically, as it occurs in both men and women.

The issue of estrogen and heart disease is crucial to an understanding of the Greatest Experiment, because it is a clear example of how women were misled about hormones. While it can be demonstrated that hormone therapy treats hot flashes and helps maintain bone mass (although perhaps not at an advisable risk), it was never *proven* to be helpful in preventing or treating heart disease. The science was just not there. Doctors did not have much right to be shocked when serious clinical data showed no connec-tion between drug and disease, since they never had any solid, compre-hensive data to the contrary. But for "reasons not fully understood," menopausal and postmenopausal women were led to believe otherwise. For that, all women have the right to be truly, righteously mad.

HEALTH IN THE BALANCE: UNDERSTANDING BONES, BONE LOSS, AND NEW METHODS OF OSTEOPOROSIS PREVENTION AND TREATMENT

In treating osteoporosis, a condition that inspires fear in the hearts of millions of elderly women and men, it is important to first determine what the condition is. When we ask, "What is osteoporosis?" it becomes clear that most people, including the doctors who aspire to prevent and treat it, have only a vague understanding of the condition. As Dr. Susan Love writes in her *Hormone Book*, "The definition of osteoporosis has gone through many permutations over the years."

For most physicians, an osteoporotic patient is identified through a series of bone mineral density (BMD) and bone measurement tests. The National Osteoporosis Foundation recommends BMD testing for all women sixty-five and older, as well as for all postmenopausal women who have had a bone fracture, have been taking hormones for a prolonged period of time, or have additional risk factors (other than menopause) for osteoporosis. The score is expressed as a standard deviation above or below the bone density of a normal young adult of the same sex. The more negative the number, the greater the risk of fracture. A patient with a BMD score between 1 and −1 is considered normal, while a patient with a score between −1 and −2.5 is considered to have osteopenia, or diminished bone. A score lower than −2.5 marks the point at which physicians say a patient has osteoporosis. Using this definition, it is estimated that more than 20 percent of postmenopausal women have osteoporosis, although some researchers estimate the number to be closer to 50 percent.

During the 1990s, the immediate response of the medical community to a diagnosis of osteoporosis or osteopenia was to put the patient on a hormone-therapy regimen. (Indeed, estrogen was suggested as a possible preventive treatment for postmenopausal osteoporosis as early as 1941.) By 1975, the annual number of estrogen prescriptions written in the United States was nearly double the numbers written in 1966, and Premarin, the country's leading estrogen product, became one of the top five prescription medications in the country. Although during this period, estrogen was marketed heavily for treatment of the psychological discomforts of menopause, keeping bones strong was an important part of its purported youth-giving properties.

Historian Elizabeth Siegel Watkins writes, however, that "estrogen turned from hero to villain" in December 1975, when four studies offered conclusive evidence that estrogen users were five to fourteen times more likely to get endometrial cancer than were nonusers. The finding coincided with the work of the movement to educate women about their bodies and their health while exposing ways in which the medical and pharmaceutical establishments had historically exploited them. These women's health activists suggested that doctors, scientists, and drug companies had not been acting in the best interests of their patients, and studies linking estrogen to endometrial cancer supported this thesis. Under pressure from grassroots activists as well as the FDA, Premarin altered its advertising claims to include only menopausal symptoms such as hot flashes, night sweats, and vaginal dryness as indications for the drug. Within five years, the number of annual estrogen prescriptions fell by 50 percent, and the pharmaceutical industry began a frantic scramble to save what had been one of its most popular drugs. It found salvation in aggressively promoting hormone therapy as the preferred treatment for osteoporosis.

Siegel Watkins writes that in the begining of the 1980s, "the preventative effect of estrogen on osteoporosis received more and more attention and endorsement." Even earlier, in 1978, Wyeth-Ayerst, the manufacturer of Premarin, resumed advertising the prevention of osteoporosis as a major use for the drug. A flurry of new research studies, government consensus reports, and pharmaceutical ballyhooing soon supported the ability of estrogens to treat thinning bones. The seal of approval became official in 1986, when the FDA announced that it considered estrogen effective for treating postmenopausal osteoporosis. Then, in the early 1990s, the renewed estrogen wave gained even more momentum when observational data suggested that hormone therapy could reduce the risk of heart disease as well.

Given the possible health problems that compromised bone density can lead to, it is not surprising that millions have flocked to their doctors in terror of skeletal thinning. As the National Women's Health Network observes in its recent book, *The Truth About Hormone Therapy*, "Scaring women about their bone strength has become a burgeoning industry. Ads depict women slumped in wheelchairs and urge us to 'talk to our doctors about osteoporosis before it's too late.' Free bone mineral density tests are offered to see 'how much we've lost.' "

Despite the scoring mentioned earlier, there are, at present, no internationally accepted guidelines for the use of bone density in trying to assess risk for osteoporosis. Definitions of the condition are changeable, and the way the medical community establishes the contemporary definition is the result of a negotiated political process. As Dr. Love explains, "Current definitions" of osteoporosis are "agreed upon by a national consensus panel of medical experts"—panels that are "generally funded by government agencies, sometimes with the help of drug companies." A situation in which the very people profiting from osteoporosis's status as a disease are the ones defining it as such presents a difficult ethic to be sure. As NWHN writes: "Behind all this great national concern is an entire industry that stands to profit from turning a risk factor into a disease. And profit they do, as an entire generation of women are being forced to take hormones."

So what difference does it make if osteoporosis is defined as a disease or as a risk factor? Well, risk, for example, is one factor among many that may or may not increase your chances of a certain hazardous outcome—just as long-term use of birth control pills may increase your risk of breast cancer but is certainly not the only, or even the primary, determining factor. According to NWHN, "Although preventing osteoporosis is one of the things we should be trying to do to prevent fractures, it is not—as the pharmaceutical industry would have us believe—the only thing."

It has become abundantly clear in the past several years that estrogen has not lived up to its reputation and that its multiple dangers make the decision to use estrogen a serious one. Not to be dismissed are the new drugs such as bisphosphonates that are giving patients other options for maintaining—and possibly enhancing—bone density. However, it is also important to consider nonmedical options for strengthening bones and preventing falls.

This is a bewildering time for woman who fear fractures, because the definition of osteoporosis is slowly starting to shift again. At a millennial National Institutes of Health Consensus Conference, it was decided to officially return to discussing osteoporosis as a risk factor. In these days of increasing retreat from estrogen as the gold standard for treatment of menopause and osteoporosis, alternatives—in particular, balance- and strength-training exercise—are becoming frontline defenses against breaking bones.

The immediate diagnosis and treatment of osteoporosis as a disease is gradually giving way to discussion of fracture prevention. At the same time, the complicated role of nutrition in bone health is being emphasized. Calcium, which has always been acknowledged as a primary factor in bone health, is increasingly important, given the uncertainty about drug treatments. Finally, in seeking nonmedical alternatives for osteoporosis, we must consider factors in addition to natural menopause that seem to play a role in declining bone health.

THE BIG DEAL ABOUT BONES

The health and safety of bones is a major concern for everybody, regardless of age. Bones are responsible for protecting vulnerable organs, including the brain, heart, and lungs. They help us maintain an upright posture and facilitate locomotion. Recent studies have even suggested a possible correlation between low bone density and serious medical conditions such as stroke.

However, methods of diagnosing osteoporosis, primarily by BMD measurement, are deeply flawed. They take into account bone density alone, which is only one component of total bone health. Bone quality, an equally important factor in how likely bones are to break, cannot be quantitatively measured. Because of this, the medical community has for years used bone density as a proxy for quality, erroneously seeing the two as one and the same. Such conflation and simplification is a common medical practice. For example, for years, doctors told patients to fear all cholesterol, yet we now know that some cholesterol is harmful while other cholesterol is beneficial to health. Understanding bones is a similarly complicated issue and must be addressed as such.

Here are some reasons, other than osteoporosis, why bones break:

- Lack of lean muscle mass (making us less strong and more likely to fall)
- Use of long-acting tranquilizers, antidepressants, and other drugs
- Ill-fitting footwear (making one more likely to fall)
- Being thin (giving the bones less natural padding)
- Removal of ovaries, especially before natural menopause
- Cigarette smoke, alcoholism
- Use of cortisone and other steroid drugs
- Lack of handrails and proper lighting in public spaces

In order to understand bone health, we must first understand what bones are. Most people think of them as solid, dead supports, like the beams that hold up their houses. Dr. Lila Wallis explains that "bone is not a dead tissue. It is a living organ. Throughout our life, from minute to minute it undergoes constant remodeling: it is being formed and resorbed, rebuilt and demolished." When stress is put on a bone, the body creates more bone to handle it. If a bone lies dormant, the body has no reason to create new bone and slowly begins to resorb the existing bone, causing it to become thin and brittle.

Like muscle building, bone building requires weight bearing and physical activity. Just as when we are young, we shape and tone our muscles at the gym, so as we age must we be diligent about building our bones. To take the analogy one step further: As is true in building muscle, no supplement or drug can safely and effectively replace actual physical activity as a means of building bone. As Dr. Wallis writes: "The bone responds positively both to gravity as well as to the local stresses. Absence of gravity and/or local stresses initiates bone resorption automatically. This cycle of bone turnover—linked resorption/rebuilding—goes on until the day we die."

There are two types of bone: the cortical and the cancellous. Cortical bone is compact and strong. It makes up most of the long bones of our extremities and covers other flat and cubical bones. Cancellous bone, which is softer, is present on the inside of all bones. It consists of bone spicules (small needlelike structures) and plates that connect to form a network. With osteoporotic bone loss, the spicules and plates shrink and their interconnection is destroyed, seriously weakening the bone.

When we refer to osteoporotic fractures, we are talking about a wide variety of possible injuries, including fracture of the spinal vertebrae, the hips, the wrists, the ribs, and the pelvis. Dr. Wallis explains that of all these fractures, those "of the hip are the most serious, leading to disability and death in about one-fifth of all hip fracture sufferers within six months."

The fact that all fractures are not created equal is crucially important when analyzing the data on fracture rates presented in various studies. While 20 percent of hip fractures are eventually fatal, it has been found that women who experience wrist fractures live, on average, longer than those who do not experience them. The difference may exist because women who get wrist fractures may be more active and healthier, the fractures themselves a result of their activity. As the *New England Journal of Medicine's Health Facts* points out, "Researchers aren't taking into account the fact that wrist, hip, and vertebral fractures are all very different and have different health implications. A hip fracture, especially in the frail elderly, may put a woman in bed for an extended period of time, increasing her chances for pneumonia, pulmonary embolism, and death. Vertebral fractures may or may not be painful and are rarely life-threatening.

A wrist fracture does not compromise mobility." Also to be taken into account is that 60 percent of bone strength and structure is inherited, and no amount of treatment, drug or otherwise, can alter genetics.

EXERCISE AS PREVENTION AND TREATMENT

After we have accepted that we can't change our genetic heritage, what is the best way to go about treating and protecting bones? How, for example, can we empower our bone quality, which is a more elusive factor in bone strength than is bone density. Take as an analogy a fine porcelain plate that may survive being dropped while a piece of common garden pottery might shatter. The reason: Despite less density, the micro architecture of the fine plate has greater tensile strength and elasticity.

So it is with bones: The stronger our bones, the better our chances of not suffering fractures from falls and accidents. Pat Crawshaw, a Canadian osteoporosis specialist, writes of a growing awareness that "much of the age-induced increased risk of fracture is an artifact of diminished muscle strength and balance, and there is increasing evidence that though exercise doesn't increase bone mineral density, it greatly reduces fracture rate."

There are three major types of exercise that help prevent fractures: balance training (which prevents falls), strength training (which builds bone), and aerobic training (which builds muscle). Dr. Laura Toshi, an orthopedic surgeon who consults for the federal government's Office of Research on Women's Health, recommends balance training as the number one strategy against fractures.

One of the safest and most effective methods of balance training has been found to be tai chi, a traditional Chinese conditioning exercise.

There are well over a hundred forms of tai chis consisting of the repertoire, but fall prevention in the elderly consists of a limited number of movements that can be easily mastered. For centuries, the elderly in China have gone to their local parks in early morning to practice, bringing with them their pet birds, which they place in nearby trees while they themselves go through the graceful, dancelike motions characteristic of the regimen. Tai chi not only teaches balance but strengthens the mind and enhances the mind-body connection. It promotes the development of relaxed breathing patterns, natural posture alignment, and clear mental focus.

Dr. Joseph M. Lane of Cornell University and Lisa Langer explain the history of tai chi:

Originating in China during the Yuan Dynasty (1279–1368 A.D.), tai chi is based on the Chinese nature philosophy of Taoism, a timeless philosophy whose concepts include harmony with oneself and the environment, gentleness of flow both internally and externally, and natural change and transformation of all things in the universe. The Chinese concept of "chi" or energy is essential to the understanding and practice of tai chi, and may best be understood as one's intrinsic energy and vitality, qualities with which we are born and may develop fully within the course of our lives.

Tai chi is particularly effective because it meets two of the three criteria for preventing fractures: It has been evaluated scientifically in terms of its benefit for the achievement of balance—thus preventing falls—and the enhancement of one's cardiovascular system, and in both of these areas it has been shown to be effective. As Lane and Langer explain, "A number of rigorous scientific studies have now concluded that tai chi will improve multiple parameters of balance and sway, and decrease falls." They add that, unlike drug treatments, "the benefits of tai chi persist long after tai chi has been terminated."

These are the five basic principles of tai chi:

I. Relax. *This principle is achieved through deep lower-abdominal breathing.*

2. Separate yin from yang. *This principle is best described as the shifting of one's weight from side to side — from the right and left sides of the body during movement. The yang side is full and weight bearing and the yin side is empty and non–weight bearing.*

3. Maintain a straight back. *When the back is aligned and maintained in a straight, upright but nonrigid position, postural control is more easily achieved. One's muscular structure functions effectively, with reduction in excessive tone and the improvement of body awareness.*

4. Turn the waist. *This is the position from which all tai chi movement starts. Turning the waist increases range of motion of the pelvis, lower back, and hips. An overall decrease in muscular rigidity in these areas improves one's balance. (For those with osteoporosis or weakened bones, it is important that this twisting be relaxed. Exercises with strong twisting motions and motions that put pressure on the spine should be avoided.)*

5. "Beautiful lady's wrists." *This refers to the position in which the wrist joint is held during tai chi practice. The wrist is held in the neutral position, without a sharp angle at the joint. This is the style in which the entire body is held while doing tai chi.*

The importance of building muscle as well as bone through weight training and cardiovascular activity is illustrated in a 1996 Mayo Clinic study, which found that strong back muscles played a role in preventing fracture in women with osteoporosis. Researchers measured back strength and bone density of thirty-six women aged forty-seven to eighty-four with osteoporosis. The women with the stronger back muscles had fewer fractures and were less stooped. According to the article, back-strengthening exercises could be as simple as "sitting in a chair and squeezing the shoulders together at the back; the other involves lifting the torso slightly off the floor while lying tummy down." Increased muscle in the back both alleviates pressure on the spine and creates better posture.

For patients with delicate bones, knowing which exercises to avoid is as important as knowing which to practice. It is a good rule to avoid any exercise that concentrates on *forcefully* bending and twisting the spine. Marjorie Bissinger writes: "Individuals with osteoporosis and osteopenia should avoid any exercises that increase forward bending or rounding of the spine." These exercises include sit-ups, toe touches, and the use of exercise equipment that applies flexion forces (some abdominal machines). Forward-bending exercises have been found to increase the incidence of spinal fractures in women who have osteoporosis.

The benefit of various exercises can be maximized by observing a few principles: Marjorie Bissinger writes that "targeting areas most prone to fractures" can help to build up strength where it is most needed, and allows exercise to be site specific. As a person progresses in her exercise regimen, it can be a good idea to increase resistance levels. Finally, although some exercises show benefits that continue once someone ceases performing them, it is best to maintain exercise programs in order to continue to receive maximum benefit.

Nutrition and Bone Health

In this new millennium, as important scientists are backing away from using estrogen as their principal treatment for osteoporosis, there has been a decided return to natural management of osteoporosis. Exercise and calcium are once again at stage center, though calcium had never actually left the wings but rather remained there, doing the work that estrogen drugs took credit for.

A quick look at several major health publications during the 1990s, the height of estrogen myth-making, shows calcium was still recommended as a constant companion. As the May 1998 *Johns Hopkins Medical Letter* states, "Calcium plus hormone replacement therapy may be the best regimen for combating osteoporosis." The article explains that although many women think that while on hormone therapy they need not take calcium, studies in fact found marked improvement in bone density among women who supplemented estrogen with calcium. According to a report, for example, in the *University of California at Berkeley Wellness Letter* in April 1998, readers were warned: "If you're a woman on hormone replacement therapy, make sure you consume lots of calcium from food or supplements. That was the bottom line of a review of 31 studies on the subject in the *American Journal of Clinical Nutrition* [AJCN]." Similar items appeared in several other publications, usually as part of a series of brief summaries encapsulating the basic information rather than giving specific study details or analysis.

One health publication, *The New England Journal of Medicine's Health News,* chose to address the AJCN findings in its "Physician's Perspective" column. In this monthly feature, a controversial study or health finding is explained, and then a doctor chosen by *Health News* analyzes it.

In this case, the appointed doctor wrote that "women who took estrogen and an average of 1,183 mg of calcium a day had almost triple the amount of new bone as women who took estrogen and less than 600 mg of calcium a day." This information is quickly tempered by the analysis of Dr. Bess Dawson-Hughs, who assures readers that "numerous studies have shown that calcium alone doesn't build bone, but only slows bone loss. Estrogen or calcitonin alone builds small amounts of bone." Dr. Dawson-Hughs, who is senior scientist and chief of the Calcium and Bone Metabolism Laboratory at the USDA Human Nutrition Research Center on Aging in Boston (a lab that acknowledges "foundation" and "industry" support on its website), is quick to dismiss any notion that calcium alone might be responsible for increased bone gain. However, she also offers no data from specific studies to support her contention that calcium alone doesn't build bone. None of the health newsletters that carried the "calcium improves HRT" story provided comparative data on calcium and exercise versus calcium and hormone therapy. The message from health newsletters was clear: Estrogen is the agent of bone building and calcium improves it, not vice versa—but the message may not be accurate after all.

Supplements other than calcium also may play a role in maintaining good bone health. Vitamin D, for one, helps the body absorb calcium and maintain bone strength. Its primary source has traditionally been sunlight. Yet as people try increasingly to protect their skin against the sun by wearing sunscreen and staying out of strong sunlight, they also block the production of vitamin D. Milk is another source of D, but a person would have to consume huge quantities of milk to get enough of the vitamin D.

In 1998, researchers at Massachusetts General Hospital in Boston discovered that 57 percent of a population of adults being studied, age eighteen to ninety, were deficient in vitamin D, a finding upsetting in part because of the interrelationship between calcium and vitamin D. If the

American people are not, as the article suggests, "getting their daily recommended amounts of vitamin D," then they aren't, by extension, absorbing the optimum amount of calcium they could be. The suggested daily dose of vitamin D was recently raised to as much as 800 IU.

Another dietary change that can positively affect bone health is to increase the consumption of foods rich in potassium, such as bananas, tomatoes, and orange juice. According to a May 23, 2002, study conducted by the University of California, San Francisco, potassium-rich foods help prevent osteoporosis by decreasing calcium loss.

As for the dietary elements found to have an adverse effect on bone health, you need only look to the unholy trinity of caffeine, cigarettes, and alcohol.

Different nutritional factors have a complicated and integrated effect on bone health. A reexamination of this can provide a starting place for establishing new, nondrug solutions to the problem of maintaining strong bones. But there is much to study and learn. The FDA, for example, recommends only an adequate daily calcium intake equivalent to 1,500 mg, either in diet alone or diet plus a calcium supplement, along with vitamin D to help with absorption. But there are no recommendations regarding other osteo-friendly substances.

Other Medical Factors That Can Have an Impact on Bone

Several medications are commonly prescribed that can have a profoundly negative effect on bone health. Steroids, specifically glucocorticoids such as prednisone, hydrocortisone, and dexamethasone, taken to treat serious conditions like asthma, lupus, arthritis, and Crohn's disease, are a major and rigorously documented factor in bone thinning. Bone loss from steroid use can be observed as soon as six months after initiating use.

Inhaled steroids became the standard treatment for asthmatics a little over a decade ago. At that point, it was thought that steroids posed little to no risk to bones. A National Osteoporosis Foundation brochure entitled "Stand Up to Osteoporosis: Your Guide to Staying Healthy and Independent Through Prevention and Treatment," newly revised in 1999, details the case history of a man named Jeff McMillian, whose bones were affected by the oral steroids he had taken to treat his asthma. The booklet explains that "Jeff's doctor was able to substitute the oral glucocorticoid with an inhaled form, which supposedly is confined to the bronchia and therefore has fewer bone thinning side effects." Yet an October 2001 *New England Journal of Medicine* study, which looked at 109 asthmatic women, revised that finding. The women were divided into three groups—one that didn't inhale steroids, another that took four to eight puffs a day, and a third that inhaled eight or more puffs a day. The results were unexpected and startling: Not only did inhaled steroids cause bone loss, but they specifically "caused bone loss at the hip," the most serious site of fractures. Despite such findings, the study concluded that "inhaled glucocorticoids . . . remain among the most effective and safest medications for the treatment of asthma." However, the report suggested "therapy adjustments to the lowest dose possible and periodic bone density measurements."

The September 2001 *Johns Hopkins Medical Letter: Health After 50* gives tips on taking glucocorticoids as safely as possible. It suggests determining the lowest effective dose for individual patients through trial and error in consultation with a doctor, halving higher-dose pills, and dosing only every other day. It stresses that these techniques are very effective for alleviating short-term side effects of the drugs and not particularly effective for bone health. The article notes, "Steps to protect the bones should always be taken. Everyone on long-term glucocorticoid therapy should consume 1,500 mg of calcium daily, along with 400 to 800 IU of vitamin D, and should exercise daily." Bisphosphonate drugs, calcitonin, and of course estrogen are offered as alternatives as well.

The effects from inhaled steroids for the treatment of asthma are similar to those from oral steroids taken for arthritis, estimated to be used for 30 million Americans. Steroids make bone adversely responsive to parathyroid hormone as well as to vitamin D, thus increasing bone loss. As Dr. Susan Love writes, "Taking steroids such as prednisone or cortisone for a long time is likely to decrease bone mass." It is startling to realize that such documented hazards to bone health are the product not of menopause or any other natural function but rather the result of drugs prescribed by doctors. This situation gives the pharmaceutical industry a huge leg up. Drugs they profit from cause bone loss, and drugs they also profit from in turn treat it. Talk about a win-win situation!

A June 17, 2002, study published in the *Journal of Bone and Mineral Research* raises concerns about the new generation of nonsteroidal anti-inflammatory drugs (NSAIDs)—namely Vioxx and Celebrex—which are often used to ease the pain of broken bones. Unlike older NSAIDs, such as ibuprofen and indomethacin, which prevent pain by inhibiting the Cox-1 and Cox-2 enzymes that catalyze the production of chemicals involved in inflammation and have long been known to delay the healing of broken bones by a few weeks without actually halting bone repair, the second-generation NSAIDs nearly entirely block the Cox-2 enzyme. And scientists now believe this enzyme, while associated with inflammation, is also essential in helping to form stem cells and growth factors that lead to restored bones. All of which reinforces a truism about new drugs: Their health risks can be grossly underestimated. As the National Health Network's Susan Jordan says, "The greater the action, the greater the reaction."

Dr. Gordon Guyatt, the Canadian father of "evidence-based medicine," reminds us that a certain percentage of new drugs is dangerous at any level: "Nearly 20 million Americans took one or more of the five drugs withdrawn from the market between September 1997 and September 1998"—drugs that were the worst of the worst. If a drug has major benefits and kills only a few people, it stays on the shelves, he adds. Does that mean we should stay away from new drugs? It depends, says Dr. Guyatt, "on how much they have to offer. If the new drug does provide a major advance, holding back would be a mistake. But each year only a handful of drugs represent an important step forward. If there is a tried and true drug that does the job, that is usually the one to use." Prescribers who are "evidence-based" therefore suggest that unless you urgently need a drug, it is wise to wait until it has been on the market for five years, allowing sufficient time for its side effects to be assessed.

The FDA has now placed black boxes not only on estrogen but on some of the new osteoporosis treatments that are coming to market, warning that serious side effects may occur. None of these products is to be taken lightly, nor are drugs prescribed for other purposes that can weaken our bones or make us vulnerable to falls. Tranquilizers, for example, may cause dizziness or disorientation and so make a person likely to lose balance, heightening the risk of fractures.

Another class of drugs that may be hazardous to bones are antidepressants. The October 1998 *HealthFacts* reports that there is "a two- to threefold increase in the risk of falling for the elderly treated with any type of antidepressant compared to those not given drugs." Nursing-home patients on antidepressants saw their risks of injury increase 50 to 200 percent with antidepressants. As *HealthFacts* points out, "This is an example of an all too common medical paradox: A treatment may end up causing the very problems it is designed to prevent—in this case, premature death and loss of function due to depression."

A link between the thyroid and bone loss has also been suggested. As the June 2001 edition of *Health News* reports, "Thyroid and parathyroid hormones . . . play important roles in the dynamic, ongoing process of bone formation and destruction." Certainly for many years, doctors have observed a connection between hyperthyroidism and osteoporotic fractures. The April 3, 2001, *Annals of Internal Medicine* reports that in a four-year study of 9,704 older women over sixty-five, those with hyperthyroidism faced a higher risk of new hip and spine fractures. Reporting on another study—one that compared 398 women randomly chosen from the original group with 148 who had new hip fractures and 149 who had new spine fractures during the follow-up period—*Health News* notes that "women presumed to have excessive thyroid hormone . . . were three times more likely to have a hip fracture and four times more likely to have a spine fracture" than women with normal thyroid-hormone levels.

Hypertension, or high blood pressure, is another risk factor in bone loss as documented in a 2000 study published in the *Lancet*. This study followed 3,676 women all aged seventy-three, for an average of 3.5 years. It was discovered that the women with high blood pressure lost bone mass at almost twice the rate as those with low blood pressure. Reporting on the study, Cornell University's *Women's Health Advisor* notes that its "authors hypothesize that women with hypertension may lose more calcium in their urine than do healthy women."

Then too, something as simple as a sedentary lifestyle can be a serious impediment to healthy bones. The fact that bones, when unused, tend to became thin, means that those laid up in bed can be particularly in danger of developing osteoporosis. As a 1996 study reported in *Environmental Nutrition* explains, "When you're confined to bed, whether you're recovering from a lengthy illness or just a case of the flu, your body begins losing bone after just one day," according to calcium expert Robert Heaney, M.D., of Creighton University in Omaha, Nebraska. It is interesting to reflect that even the common cold, if it is severe enough to keep you off your feet for a few days, can have a direct and immediate effect on bone density. Once you've recovered, however, an easy remedy is to diligently maintain a workout program.

Another measure that can reduce the risk of fracture if you happen to be on the slim side is to gain weight, since thin people simply don't have the padding to cushion their bones should they fall. Of course, since being heavy is associated with a host of problems, including heart disease, a healthier solution might be to add a little padding to your wardrobe. A November 23, 2000, issue of *The New England Journal of Medicine* reported that wearing hip protectors made older adults with weak bones 60 percent less likely to break a hip than those who didn't wear them. It is also a good idea to make sure that rugs are secured so that they don't slip out from under you, that furniture is not in harm's way, and that lighting is adequate.

Maintaining bone health, of course, is a process that is not just a concern of the elderly. It is best to begin early in life, long before menopause is reached. First, and most basic, young women must get adequate amounts of calcium. As I wrote in "Taking Control of Your Health," a chapter in the book *Hands On! 33 More Things Every Girl Should Know*, "A whopping 35 to 40 percent of all the bone mass you will ever have is laid down" during puberty, from about age ten to fourteen in girls. If girls at this age make sure to get the recommended 1,300 mg of calcium a day, they can go a long way toward preventing future problems. In the piece, I described how my granddaughter Sophia and I sat down and discussed how important calcium was, and established simple ways she could meet her daily requirement. I wrote: "At first Sophia was discouraged when she studied my tables on the calcium content of different foods. Reluctantly she said she'd try to drink two cups of milk each day, instead of one, which would bring her to 600 mg, or almost halfway. She brightened when she realized that instead of the second glass of milk, she could have a yogurt, and all but glowed to discover that two glasses of fortified juice would take her to 1,000 mg." Sometimes the most important contribution one can make to the prevention of osteoporosis is to educate our children to lead healthier lives and to be alert to the onset of any eating disorder before it becomes entrenched.

I'm thinking here particularly of anorexia nervosa, a disease most common in young women that can have disastrous effects on bones even years after recovering from the illness. A clinical study on the bone complications associated with such an eating disorder, presented in June 2001 at the First Joint Meeting of the International Bone and Mineral Society and the European Calcified Tissue Society, revealed that "young Danish women with anorexia nervosa and bulimia were 2 to 3 times more likely to suffer a fracture than women without such disorders." The study further revealed that anorexic young women can fail to achieve peak bone mass, which may increase risk of fracture "even more dramatically as they enter menopause."

Young women should also be aware of the side effects before deciding to go on Depo-Provera, a progesterone contraceptive given by injection that has been shown to cause bone loss in some users. In her book *The Menopause Industry*, Sandra Coney writes that "after measuring the bones of young women who had been using Depo-Provera for over five years, it was found that they had 7.5% less bone in the spine and 6.5% less bone in the hip than women who had never used the drug." The bone loss seems to result from the drug's blocking of estrogen and causing amenorrhea (the absence of menstruation).

Current findings about the dangers of hormone therapy aside, today's emphasis on preventing fractures through practical, nonmedical means generates health benefits that go far beyond their implications for bone, protecting the heart and other organs as well. These new approaches have also led scientists and doctors to reexamine the complicated nutritional balance that creates skeletal health. Thus has begun a long overdue reevaluation of old methods for treating osteoporosis and a more complete understanding of what protects bones and keeps them from breaking.

LOSING OUR MINDS TO HORMONES: THE PREMATURE PRESCRIBING OF ESTROGEN FOR ALZHEIMER'S DISEASE

Many of us can identify with the sixty-six-year-old Harvard profes- sor who forgot her classroom number when ordering a slide projector. She went directly to the office of the university's Alzheimer's specialist and asked, "Am I losing it?" Was she having a senior moment or was it something far worse? Was it Alzheimer's?

Three percent of adults ages sixty-five to seventy-four develop this dread disease, and the percentage rises as age advances. Many of us who have watched a parent or an elderly friend struggle with Alzheimer's debilitating effects live in mortal fear of someday succumbing to the same fate. As baby boomers approach the passage between middle age and senior status, there is overwhelming interest revolving around what can be done to reduce the odds of developing Alzheimer's and upping the chances of preserving memory.

It is very hard to accept the fact that little actually *can* be done, but a desire to be proactive has created a huge market for products claiming to help—products ranging from vitamin supplements to diet and exercise regimens to pharmaceuticals.

Since 1994, with the publication of a paper in the *American Journal of Epidemiology* called "Estrogen Deficiency and the Risk of Alzheimer's Disease in Women," estrogen supplementation and other hormone therapies have been promoted as a way to improve memory and stave off Alzheimer's. This despite the fact that precious little evidence has emerged that estrogen does fight the disease. So how do pharmaceutical companies continue to market the drug as a means of combating AD? By conflating normal menopausal memory problems and natural aging-associated cognitive impairment with Alzheimer's; women have been bamboozled into believing that treating the first two means preventing the last.

That we have nothing but the slimmest evidence to support any positive relationship between estrogen and the prevention of Alzheimer's is not for lack of trying. The sheer volume of scientific work that has been done on this topic in the past decade is overwhelming. Even more astounding is how many millions of dollars it has taken us to conclude that there is no good evidence that estrogen either prevents or treats Alzheimer's disease, and that as of yet, the relationship between hormones and AD is not understood.

THE CHRISTENING OF AD

Our parents did not worry about Alzheimer's. Until the 1970s and '80s, the general public wasn't really aware of it. It is hard to determine how common Alzheimer's was before the twentieth century because it wasn't until then that the disease was identified. Prior to that time, it was not plainly differentiated from the normal forgetfulness of aging, yet it seems likely that even then AD did exist as a discrete condition. In his book *The Forgetting*, David Shenk describes the senile dementia of Ralph Waldo Emerson: "At age 74, this was no longer the Ralph Waldo Emerson who had written 'Self Reliance' and 'Nature' . . . This was now a very different man, a waning crescent, caught in the middle stages of a progressive memory disorder that had ravaged his concentration and short-term memory and so dulled his perceptions that he was no longer able to understand what he read or follow a conversation."

On November 15, 1901, Dr. Alois Alzheimer, a neuropathologist in Frankfurt, interviewed a fifty-one-year-old patient named Auguste D., who exclaimed, "I have lost myself." The doctor was confused. How could such a relatively young woman be going senile?

When Auguste D. died on April 8, 1906, Alzheimer sent for her brain. When he examined it, he found that it looked as if it were infected with measles or chicken pox and was sprouting weeds. He called the crusty brown clumps "plaques" and the weedlike growths "tangles."

In 1910, Emil Kraepelin, dean of German psychiatry, named the condition identified by Dr. Alzheimer as Alzheimer's disease. For the next half century, Alzheimer's disease was acknowledged, if at all, as a rare disorder afflicting relatively young adults. Old-age dementia (and the loss or impairment of mental powers) was attributed to atherosclerosis—i.e., fatty deposits that can clog the brain.

In 1952, Dr. Meta Neumann, the curator of the Brain Bank at St. Elizabeth's Psychiatric Hospital in Washington, D.C., had an epiphany that proved Alzheimer's was not so rare as scientists had thought. Neumann was called to autopsy an elderly colleague who died without warning soon after he had "ably led a vigorous meeting with the hospital staff." His brain was severely clogged with the fatty deposits thought to cause dementia, and yet he had retained his full intellect right up to his last day. Neumann matched the physical characteristics she found in her colleague's brain with the psychiatric histories and physical characteristics of the brains of 210 people who had been diagnosed with dementia. She found that few of the brains showed sclerosis like her colleague's; rather, they had plaques and tangles. In other words, they had "Alzheimer's brains." Shenk writes: "It was not a rare disease after all."

Neumann's findings were ignored for some time, but by the 1970s, thanks to the persistence of Dr. Robert Butler at the NIH, concern over Alzheimer's was stirred and research into the disease supported. But the final leap into full public awareness didn't come until 1987 with the publication of a government report entitled *Losing a Million Minds: Confronting the Tragedy of Alzheimer's Disease and Other Dementias.* Meanwhile, in the first burst of enthusiasm, many people were misdiagnosed with AD when in fact they had dementia owing to other conditions, such as depression, thyroid disease, hypoglycemia, drug interactions, or chronic infection.

ANATOMY OF A NO-BRAINER

Today, it is claimed that Alzheimer's is the fourth leading cause of death in the United States—after heart disease, cancer, and stroke. Though there are still many unanswered questions about the exact nature of the condition, what we do know is that it is responsible for 55 percent of all dementia cases, and that it is a disorder marked by memory loss, confusion, and impaired thinking.

Alzheimer's is distinguished from other types of dementia by the way it physically changes the brain, strangling and shrinking it with plaques and tangles characteristic of the disease. In the 1980s, researchers discovered that plaques—which develop in the spaces between neurons and occur early in the disease process, sometimes as early as twenty years before symptoms appear—were largely cell debris surrounded by beta-amyloid, a protein that is a by-product of a larger protein involved in cell membrane function. Beta-amyloid is secreted by cells throughout the body but is produced in especially large amounts in the brain.

Tangles are composed of dying nerve cells made of the protein tau. The internal support structure of nerve cells depends on tau working normally. In people with Alzheimer's, threads of tau go through compositional change that causes them to twist, eventually strangling and killing neurons. Tangles seem to develop later in the disease progression, but scientists are still unsure whether that is true.

It takes an average of eight years to erase the brain, regressing a person to a state that resembles infancy. It is, by all accounts, excruciating for caregivers as well as for those suffering from the disease. In a *New Yorker* article entitled "My Father's Brain," novelist Jonathan Franzen describes the harrowing experience of watching his own father deteriorate from the disease. He writes: "My father was an intensely private person, and privacy for him had the connotation of keeping the shameful content of one's interior life out of public sight. Could there have been a worse disease for him than Alzheimer's? In its early stages, it worked to dissolve the social connection that had saved him from the worst of his depressive isolation. In its later stages, it robbed him of the sheathing of adulthood, the means to hide the child inside him. I wish he'd had a heart attack instead."

SCIENCE BY PRESS RELEASE

The prescribing of hormone therapy for Alzheimer's disease exploits this painful situation and is an example of gender-based drug marketing at its most blatant. It relies on the running together of two unrelated memory problems: normal menopausal "mind" lapses—which are often temporary but nonetheless upsetting—and Alzheimer's, as if the first can lead to the second, a claim for which there is no scientific evidence. Promoting estrogen as prevention against Alzheimer's is a classic example of "science by press release," a practice whereby essential information is deliberately omitted. Just as some doctors conceal that the most dramatic changes in bone mass are shown to occur in castrated women, they may also fail to explain that the women who feel sure their brains are benefiting from estrogen are generally those in menopause who have experienced the normal phenomenon of memory problems. As one woman described what she called her brain fog: "I stammered, I stuttered, I misread words. It's as if the coordination between my eyes and the rest of me just didn't connect. I found myself searching for the most basic one- or two-syllable words whereas I previously was extremely articulate. For a smart-ass like myself, this process was terribly frustrating."

Such trouble organizing and expressing ideas can challenge a woman's self-image. A friend explains that "I can look up and down a bookshelf for ages without finding the title I want, and it's right in front of me. I must say, I am profoundly 'hurt' by this. . . . Reading, writing, discussing, finding the perfect word within our elegant language—all these things were my idea of having a good time. Now what? If I lose my health insurance because my brain no longer functions well enough to hold down a job, that will surely shorten my life!"

Many women feel they would do almost anything to avoid or rectify these problems, making it easy for the drug companies to hook them on hormone therapy.

One woman who went on estrogen said that the "deciding factor for me in trying hormone therapy was brain function—I was losing mine! My memory was really, really bad. I spent more time going in circles than I did accomplishing anything. Sometimes I forgot what I was saying in the middle of a sentence and had this crazy inability to understand the spoken word. I was fine with anything in print or on a screen, but things people said to me sometimes sounded like gobbledygook. That was *very* scary."

The belief that hormones can help menopausal women with memory and concentration is not totally unfounded. There have been studies for some years now that suggest a relationship between estrogen and cognitive function. The connection, however, has been largely undefined and overstated. A study published in 2000, dealing with postmenopausal estrogen and progestin use and cognitive change in older Japanese American women, set out to test both the connection between estrogen and cognition and the potential difference that estrogen alone might make as opposed to an estrogen/progestin combination pill. The conclusion: Both estrogen and progestin seemed to have a beneficial effect on cognition. However, the report on the study steered scrupulously clear of making any outsized claims, being careful to note that the benefit of hormones on cognition was "modest" and "the clinical significance of these modest differences . . . is quite uncertain. Data from long-term randomized trials are required before applying this information to the clinical setting."

A later study, printed in the December 2001 edition of *Fertility and Sterility*, found that long-term postmenopausal hormone therapy did have a slight beneficial effect on women's nonverbal memory and attention. Comparing test scores (including those for memory, verbal fluency, executive functioning, concentration, and attention) of postmenopausal women sixty years and older who had and had not been treated with hormones, a team of scientists from the University of Michigan Hospital and Health Center in Ann Arbor concluded that women who used hormone therapy performed better on prefrontal and executive function tests but not on the others. They emphasized again that the benefit was "slight," noting that "further longitudinal studies appear warranted to assess both the specificity of these findings to those cognitive domains and to determine whether the findings are consistent across socioeconomic groups and educational levels."

Some nine months earlier, the March 21, 2001, issue of *JAMA* published an analysis of studies, performed by Dr. Erin S. Leblanc at the Oregon Health Sciences University in Portland, of the effects of hormone therapy on various memory problems. The article concluded that "in women with menopausal symptoms, HRT may have specific cognitive effects." Women who had experienced menopausal symptoms such as severe hot flashes and trouble sleeping were shown on hormones to have improved verbal memory, vigilance, reasoning, and motor speed. The analysis added, however, that for women without menopausal symptoms, there seemed to be little or no benefit from hormone therapy. One possible explanation for these findings is that estrogen products do effectively treat hot flashes, so that for women who haven't been able to sleep or function because of them, relief can lead to an increased ability to concentrate and think. In other words, the studies' positive conclusions about memory may be the by-product of estrogen's effect on other symptoms rather than a direct effect on the brain.

Women who go on hormone therapy programs, without symptoms, often see little to no effect on cognitive functioning. But sometimes the opposite is true. As one such woman said: "I was put on HRT by my gynecologist and I became a medical basket case. Finally I saw a neuropath who 'knew' what my symptoms were before I told him. He said he sees a lot of women with symptoms caused by perimenopause, birth control pills, and HRT. Some of the specifics he talked about were head pains, body pains, numbness of extremities, confusion, depression, fatigue, not being able to think clearly. And my favorite personal symptom—speech problems. I could not articulate, lost words, couldn't finish sentences. My case was extreme, but now that I've stopped HRT, I'm better." In April 1999, *JAMA* published the results of a Yale University study that found that although the brain-activity patterns of women on estrogen more closely resembled those of premenopausal women, there was no difference in memory test scores.

An *American Journal of Epidemiology* study from October 2001 further found no consistent change in cognition test scores between women who did and did not take estrogen. Conducted by Dr. Suzana Alves de Moraes and colleagues from Johns Hopkins University Bloomberg School of Public Health, the study collected data on 2,859 women, ages forty-eight to sixty-seven, who had their cognitive functioning tested twice by a battery of exams given between 1990 and 1998. The researchers wrote that their findings "would seem to indicate that, at least for women in the age range included in the study, use of estrogen replacement therapy is not associated with age-related cognitive declines."

Finally, among the papers published in the February 2003 issue of the AMA's *Archives of Neurology* were two dealing with estrogens—one examining the effects of Premarin on cognitive functioning and the other assessing the effects on memory of estradiol produced by the body. The first, conducted by researchers at the University of California at San Diego, investigated women with diagnosed AD, all of whom had undergone hysterectomies and thus could be given Premarin alone. Half of those on Premarin took the standard dose of 0.625 mg and the other half took a higher dose of 1.25. Researchers tracked the change in hormone levels as well as periodically administering several different tests for cognitive functioning. Hormone levels increased fourfold in women on the 0.625 dose and eightfold in those on the 1.25 dose. But there were no significant differences in cognitive functioning nor in other neuropsychological measures, compared to the women on placebo, either at two months or twelve months into the study. Similar to the effects of pharmaceutical estrogens, higher natural levels of estradiol do not help older women—or men—perform any better on memory tests, as the second study showed. To the contrary, this study, conducted in the Netherlands, found that women with higher total estradiol levels had poorer memory performance and less hippocampal matter (the hippocampus being the part of the brain responsible for memory). In men, however, there was no association observed between estradiol levels and hippocampal matter, but a trend emerged that linked higher levels of total estradiol with poorer memory performance. According to the researchers, "Our data do not support the hypothesis that higher natural levels of estrogen are associated with better memories." (In contrast to the Netherlands volunteers, who were all elderly people "with no dementia," the volunteers receiving Premarin in the San Diego study all had Alzheimer's—which does impose limitations on the study, because asking women with degenerative memory disease to recall if they've taken their medication is not the best way to collect information.)

BANG THE DRUM SOFTLY

Whatever effect hormone treatments may have on menopausal memory loss, they have no proven effect at all in preventing or treating Alzheimer's disease and dementia, despite the fact that the attempt to establish positive connection got off to a promising start. In 1994, a study of women from the Leisure World retirement community in Southern California announced that those who had taken hormones were a third less likely to develop Alzheimer's disease, the risk falling as the estrogen dosage increased. The study received a massive amount of press; coupled with findings about hormones and osteoporosis in the 1980s, and hormones and heart disease, a new estrogen renaissance kicked into highest gear. Much neglected— one might say "censored"—was a similar study reported on in *JAMA* in May 1993 that found those who took estrogen were more likely to have died of Alzheimer's than were nonusers.

An August 17, 1996, article in the *Lancet* reported that in a five-year study of 1,124 older women, Columbia University researchers discovered that only 5.8 percent of those who took estrogen developed Alzheimer's, compared to 16.3 percent of those who did not, reducing the risk of contracting AD by 87 percent. But in evaluating the study, the *Harvard Health Letter* noted: "A major limitation . . . , however, is how it was conducted: the scientists interviewed the women about postmenopausal estrogen use but had no way of verifying their answers. The resulting information is probably not as reliable as data gathered in a controlled clinical trial, where groups are assigned to different treatments and then carefully watched over time," adding that "the investigation did not look at the most beneficial doses of estrogen, the best formulation or how long HRT needs to be taken." Dr. John Growdon, a professor of neurology at Harvard Medical School, went on to caution readers that "it is probably not a good idea to start HRT solely to prevent Alzheimer's until more information is available."

Another headline-grabbing report lauded as having "tipped the balance in favor of estrogen" was the Baltimore Longitudinal Study of Aging, a sixteen-year study, the results of which were published in the June 1997 issue of *Neurology*. It found that taking estrogens reduced the risk of developing Alzheimer's by approximately 50 percent. Again, health specialists were cautious, reporting that this study, like those before it, was "observational . . . and as such, not ideal. Unlike randomized controlled trials, in which the participants are assigned to follow one course or another and are likely to have similar characteristics, observational studies offer no assurance that the women in both groups began the trial on equal footing."

Despite reveling in so-called positive findings about estrogen and Alzheimer's, scientists found themselves unable to explain how the hormone prevented the disease. They theorized that, like its protective effect on the heart (which was later disproved), perhaps estrogen kept the brain young by shielding existing neurons and encouraging further neuronal growth. The more exposure to estrogen one has, the theory posited, the more consistently one's cognitive abilities would survive.

This hypothetical relationship between estrogen and the brain was challenged in March 2001, when a Dutch study set out to document whether a longer reproductive period, which implies a longer exposure to estrogen, was associated with a lower risk of Alzheimer's. After looking at a population of 3,601 women aged fifty-five and older over the course of ten years, the authors of the study determined that their findings did "not support the hypothesis that a longer reproductive period reduces risk of dementia." In fact, women with longer reproductive periods had a slightly increased risk of developing the disease. Newsletters that relied at least partially on drug company money were quick to add spin on the study, noting that while "natural estrogen" didn't seem to protect against Alzheimer's, "ERT might."

More bad news on estrogen and the prevention of Alzheimer's came in March 2001 via the *Archives of Neurology*. Scientists attempting to resolve conflicting findings about HRT's capacity to reduce Alzheimer's risk looked at several communities of women in the United Kingdom. They concluded that "the use of ERT in women after the onset of menopause was not associated with a reduced risk of developing Alzheimer's disease."

Findings about estrogen as a preventative measure are clearly inconsistent, but findings about estrogen as an Alzheimer's treatment are almost nonexistent.

In November 1996, less than two years after the Leisure World study popularized estrogen for Alzheimer's prevention, a study was presented that looked at the effect of estrogen on twelve women with Alzheimer's. Scientists found that after eight weeks, the estrogen group performed twice as well on tests as the group not taking estrogen. Once treatment stopped, the benefits diminished, but didn't disappear entirely. Analyzing the study, *The New England Journal of Medicine Health News* commented that "because the study was so small, it's too soon to say whether hormone therapy might be a useful treatment for Alzheimer's," particularly given the fact that estrogen "when used alone as in this study, promotes cancer of the uterus and may increase the risk of breast cancer."

The February 23, 2000, *Journal of the American Medical Association* reported a study in which researchers randomly placed approximately 100 women with Alzheimer's disease on high-dose estrogen, low-dose estrogen, and a placebo. The participants had an average age of seventy-five and all had had hysterectomies. The study, led by Ruth Mulnard of the University of California at Irvine, found that while estrogen improved mental functioning after two months, it did not prevent decline after one year. In fact, the estrogen patients actually showed decline on the Clinical Dementia Rating Scale (CDR) versus those receiving placebo.

Gradually doctors were forced to admit that the outlook for treating Alzheimer's with hormones was bleak. Dr. Kristine Yaffe, an estrogen researcher at the University of California, admitted in 2001 at the annual meeting of the American Association for Geriatric Psychiatrists that "we are less optimistic that estrogen can be used as a treatment for Alzheimer's," but insisted "there is more exciting data on whether estrogen can be used against longtime decline and development of the disease."

After the halting of WHI trials, Dr. Diana Petitti of Kaiser Permanente observed in a *JAMA* editorial that "prospective observational studies continue to suggest that ERT might protect against cognitive decline and the development of dementia. Data on ERT and HRT to prevent cognitive decline and dementia are not consistent, however, and randomized trials of estrogen in the treatment of Alzheimer's disease show no evidence of benefit."

Another study, by Sudha Seshadri et al., reported in the March 2001 *Archives of Neurology*, drew on a United Kingdom research database of about 220,000 women, the largest study of Alzheimer's and estrogen to date. The conclusion: "The use of ERT in women after the onset of menopause was not associated with a reduced risk of developing Alzheimer's disease."

So given how little evidence there is for using hormones to ward off *or* treat Alzheimer's, how is it that a virtual cottage industry was built to use them for just that? The story encompasses science, health newsletters, and other major sources of medical information to equate normal cognitive problems with Alzheimer's disease, a confusion that occurs on many levels, from scientists who use data on one type of memory loss to hypothesize on the other without consistent differentiation, to newsletters (many of which receive drug company dollars) that blatantly confuse one finding with another.

A further distinction should be made between mild cognitive impairment, a clinically defined level of memory loss that is associated with early stages of Alzheimer's disease, and the menopausal memory problems associated with normal aging. According to the *Archives of Neurology*, mild cognitive impairment is a "transitional state between the cognitive changes of normal aging and Alzheimer's disease, in which persons experience memory loss to a greater extent than one would expect for age, yet they do not meet currently accepted criteria for clinically probable Alzheimer's disease." Research has indicated that a certain percentage of individuals with mild cognitive impairment develop Alzheimer's disease, and unlike menopausal or normal memory loss, there seems to be evidence to support a connection between the two. A May 1, 2001, article published in *Neurology* states that people with mild cognitive impairment have about triple the risk of developing Alzheimer's disease. When studies discuss cognitive decline, they are not necessarily talking about mild cognitive impairment; they are usually talking about decreased scores on memory tests.

I found that language is often used to confuse data on cognitive impairment with that specifically on Alzheimer's. One *Johns Hopkins Medical Letter* described the findings of the Proceedings of the National Academy of Science by noting estrogen "might" help improve memory. This weak finding on the role of HRT in slowing cognitive decline is quickly extended to include Alzheimer's: "estradiol stimulated the growth of nerve pathways in cells from a region of the brain associated with the progression of Alzheimer's disease." The finding here was on estrogen and cognitive ability. By suggesting that these findings were in "the same region of the brain as Alzheimer's," they connect the two in the reader's mind. However, unless there is data to suggest a connection, it is irresponsible to infer that the solution to one problem will necessarily cure the other.

Here is the essence of the estrogen experiment. For forty years drug companies, scientists and researchers have been playing carrot-and-stick with women's lives. They hold out poorly substantiated claims for estrogen's health benefits, which buys them time as they try to develop the proof to back up the claims. But the fact remains that after all these years, and with countless deaths attributable to estrogen via cancers, cardiovascular complications, blood clots, and other health problems, including asthma and gallbladder disease, the evidence isn't there. If the data is there, women must demand to see it before agreeing to put more pills into our bodies.

Some recent studies have focused on progesterone and testosterone as Alzheimer's treatments instead of estrogen alone. Again, the facts just aren't there, so women should be wary about these claims, too.

So if estrogen is a dangerous and unproved option for staving off or treating Alzheimer's, what can a smart meno-babe do if she wants to keep her brain functioning in top form? The best strategy is to educate yourself about AD and to stay mentally and physically active. In chapter 13, I stressed the importance of using our bones lest we lose them. The brain is in some ways similar and may benefit from staying active in community organizations, reading novels, doing crosswords, traveling. Dr. Robert S. Wilson and his colleagues at Rush Presbyterian–St. Luke's Medical Center in Chicago studied 801 elderly patients in the Religious Orders Study, an ongoing study of aging and Alzheimer's disease, to test the hypothesis that frequent participation in cognitive activities is associated with reduced risk of developing the disease. On average, participants reporting more frequent activity were 47 percent less likely to develop Alzheimer's.

For the menopausal woman worried about her memory, realizing that her daily memory struggles are not necessarily the first step down the road to Alzheimer's is reassuring, but it still leaves her with the problem of how to curb the current disruptive problems. Realizing that such problems are probably temporary may be a first step. In the meantime, exercising regularly is one simple drug-free thing a woman can do to improve her memory. In a 1999 paper at the proceedings of the National Academy of Science, Fred Gage and other researchers at the Salk Institute presented information suggesting that exercise may actually stimulate neuronal growth. Cardiovascular exercise increases blood flow, and by extension the flow of oxygen, to the brain, which can only be beneficial.

Also, talking to family members about the changes and hardships experienced during menopause may be helpful in getting through the transition. It lets people in your life know that you are undergoing major changes. Being honest with others and patient with yourself will take a weight off your mind in a manner no pill can do.

Another strategy for coping with the fear of Alzheimer's is to remember that Alzheimer's is only one in a variety of causes of memory loss and dementia. As the *Mount Sinai School of Medicine Focus on Healthy Aging* points out, "Dementia can be a symptom, sometimes temporary, of dozens of diseases and disorders. These include poisoning, reactions to medications, viral infections, malfunctioning glands, benign brain tumors, and severe nutritional deficiencies." About 10 percent of cases of dementia are due to causes that can be partially or completely reversed—the effects of a prescription medication. Vascular dementia, caused by stroke or heart attack, is the second most common cause. It is estimated that up to 42 percent of heart surgery patients suffer measurable mental deterioration during the five years after surgery, and up to 40 percent of strokes result in some degree of dementia. It can sometimes be hard to tell the difference between Alzheimer's and other forms of dementia, but vascular dementia tends to progress in a stepwise fashion, with periods of relative stability punctuated by periods of more noticeable worsening. Mental deterioration in Alzheimer's patients is more of a steady linear decline. With vascular dementia, motor troubles may be evident, whereas with Alzheimer's, symptoms are nearly all memory related. It is important to identify what kind of memory loss one is dealing with, because non-Alzheimer's dementias are often treatable and sometimes reversible.

When the dementia *is* due to Alzheimer's one potential trigger could be head injury. A study from the University of Pennsylvania School of Medicine demonstrated that mild, repetitive traumatic brain injury hastens the onset of Alzheimer's disease. They performed this experiment using mice that had been given a form of Alzheimer's disease. The mice were anesthetized, placed in a frame, and subjected to a relatively mild head impact. This trauma was repeated the next day on a select group of the mice. The mice in the second group showed a marked decline. According to the article in *Neuroscience*, "the data strongly supports previous epidemiological studies implicating traumatic brain injury as one of the most robust environmental risk factors for Alzheimer's disease."

It has long been suspected that exposure to metals may also play a role in Alzheimer's disease. This theory has been dismissed in recent years as an old wives' tale. In response to a 1997 reader question regarding a possible connection, *Environmental Nutrition* responded: "Several years ago, scientists suggested a connection between aluminum cookware and Alzheimer's disease after discovering high concentrations of aluminum in the brains of affected individuals. Today, that link has been ruled out by several well-respected health organizations" adding that aluminum in the brain is thought to be a result of the disease rather than a cause.

A more recent group of researchers at Massachusetts General Hospital have challenged this consensus, asserting that a build-up of copper and zinc in the brain causes plaques to form. According to *The Wall Street Journal*, these scientists theorize that "beta-amyloid, a naturally occurring protein, helps control metals in the brain and prevents cell damage from oxidation. . . . In Alzheimer's patients, the researchers believe beta-amyloid protein abnormally traps copper," which in turn creates hydrogen peroxide, a chemical poisonous to cells.

The New England Journal of Medicine reports that people with elevated levels of homocysteine in their blood might double their risk for Alzheimer's. Homocysteine is an amino acid normally used by the body to metabolize cells and manufacture proteins. Homocysteine levels can be reduced by increasing one's intake of folic acid and vitamins B_6 and B_{12}.

A risk factor for Alzheimer's that we can do nothing about is genetics. There is good evidence that a particular gene may be associated with elevated Alzheimer's risk. In 1995, the *Journal of the American Medical Association* announced that in a study of older adults ranging from age seventy-nine to eighty-five, 60 percent of those who tested positive for the APOE 4 protein developed Alzheimer's disease within five years. Among those not carrying the protein, only 24 percent developed the disease. Further research has associated APOE 4 with accelerated brain aging and with causing changes in nerve cells. APOE is strongly associated with early-onset Alzheimer's, which develops when people are still in their forties, fifties, or early sixties.

A multitude of new treatment strategies are currently under way for developing drugs that can attack Alzheimer's at its source, but a major problem has been that scientists are unsure which occurs first, plaques or tangles, and which are responsible for what part of the disease. Most scientists currently theorize that if the plaques can be prevented, the disease can be avoided. As the January 2002 *Harvard Health Letter* explains, "Many experts agree that [Alzheimer's is] likely to be most vulnerable to treatment at the point when bits of beta-amyloid protein start to accumulate into plaque"—and scientists are currently attempting to develop drugs that could block them.

Sadly, though, at times it seems that whenever drug companies get involved, trouble follows. The burgeoning field of Alzheimer's drug development already has a drug company embarrassment. Two years ago, Elan Corporation, a Dublin and San Francisco–based drug company, announced they were developing a potential Alzheimer's vaccine; tests were initiated in humans. In January 2002 it was announced that those trials were suspended after some patients showed signs of inflammation of the central nervous system. Despite problems, drug makers still expect the drug "to enter the market by about 2005." Unlike the case of estrogen for

Alzheimer's, at least those involved in the Elan trials are aware they are part of an experiment.

I asked the feminist Dr. Kathryn Scarbrough, a knowledgeable neuro-endocrinologist who has long followed the debate over estrogen's effect on Alzheimer's to comment on the disappointing quality of the studies to date. She said, "In my field, everyone knows you have to have a control, but the adequacy of the controls used are constantly argued. I'd attribute it to time pressures, eagerness to test a new idea, and the influence of Big Pharma," which is involved in more than 80 percent of research today.

Indeed, a study performed by Diana Petitti and her colleagues at Kaiser Permanente and published in 2002 "used a design in which we determined hormone use in the past based on computer records of pre-scriptions. We also asked women about their use of estrogen in interviews as a check." Petitti found that there was a substantial percentage of women who had dementia and denied that they had ever used estrogen, even though they had. In other words, these women forgot.

"That was a slam dunk study," says Scarbrough. "It buried former, less careful work, to the extent the evidence from former studies should no longer be considered. Which is hard to do . . . to say to yourself, 'Okay, this stuff I've believed for X years is completely wrong. I have evidence that it's wrong so I will no longer believe it.' But that is the nature of science—you have to constantly update your beliefs based on better and better informa-tion." It's also a mistake, she adds, to rely on self-reporting.

Of course, it is one thing to say that self-reporting is a possible prob-lem, it is quite another to have actual proof that the problem is causing bias. Petitti provides that proof.

CHAPTER 15

AND BEAR IN MIND . . . SWIMMING IN THE SEA OF ESTROGENS

The HRT scandal is bigger than most think. It's not just about menopausal women, like me, getting bad information from their doctors and the pharmaceutical industry for over forty years, while the federal government stood by and did nothing. The scandal is much bigger than that. We're living in a world awash with hormones.

— LYNN LANDES

In 1993, in response to pressure by breast cancer activists from Nassau and Suffolk Counties on Long Island, New York, Congress passed a law mandating the National Cancer Institute to undertake a massive study to identify "environmental and other potential risk factors contributing to the incidence of breast cancer," and to look specifically at water and air pollution, pesticides and toxic waste dumps, and other environmental agents, as possible causes of the high rates of breast cancer among Long Island women. Many of those who pressed for the Long Island Breast

Cancer Study Project hoped the study would pinpoint controllable causes of the alarming rise in breast cancer rates. Nine years and $30 million later, the project published results assessing a handful of mostly banned toxic chemicals, none of which was tied with increased breast cancer on Long Island.

In 1996, Congress adopted legislation that called for screening and testing of possible endocrine disruptors, chemicals that can interfere with the glands that regulate human fetal development, sexual maturation, reproductive function, and energy metabolism. The Environmental Protection Agency and the National Institutes of Health spent several years and a few millions of dollars investigating natural and synthetic chemicals that mimic hormones.

Shockingly, both these massive multimillion-dollar studies ignored the proverbial elephant in the room: the pharmaceutical and veterinary estrogens and other hormones that humans and animals have been eating and depositing into the environment for years—hormones that have been proven to be linked to hormone-dependent breast, uterine, ovarian, and testicular cancers. A decade earlier in 1993, Richard Sharpe of Edinburgh and Niels Skakkebaek of Copenhagen reported in *Lancet*, that "humans now live in an environment that can be viewed as a virtual sea of estrogens." In view of what was already known about the health risks of pharmaceutical hormones, the exclusion of such hormones from two supposedly serious scientific studies raises disturbing questions as to what the real point of the studies was.

Consider, for example, that in 1978 a National Task Force on diethylstilbestrol (DES) was convened by the surgeon general and the secretary of the Department of Health, Education and Welfare to address the mounting evidence of the significant health risks posed by estrogen pharmaceuticals. Federal officials asked me to serve on the DES panel, as I had written about the hormone's harmful effects in my book *Women and the Crisis in Sex Hormones*. At the task force meetings, Dr. Sidney Wolfe, founder of Public Citizen's Health Research Group, presented initial evidence that women exposed to DES during pregnancy had higher rates of breast cancer and might develop earlier and more lethal cases of the disease than other women.

In addition and above all, the task force addressed troubling concerns that had been sparked over the fate of DES daughters. At least 1.5 million women had taken DES under the mistaken notion that this would prevent miscarriages. Their daughters remained at serious risk from these brief exposures to the hormone in utero. The victims of this exposure included young women like Marilyn M., a DES daughter from Virginia who developed vaginal cancer at age fourteen, lung cancer at fifteen, and cancer in her head, hip, arms, and legs at sixteen. Two years after her initial diagnosis, Marilyn went blind and succumbed to a slow and painful death. She left behind a sister who developed adenosis, an abnormal condition in the vaginal tract thought to be a precursor to vaginal cancer.

Nine out of every ten DES daughters had deformed reproductive systems or other abnormalities that warranted careful surveillance, and half could not conceive or bear children. One in seven hundred DES daughters contracted a rare and often lethal form of cancer called adenocarcinoma. This malignancy affects glandular tissue that forms only in those whose mothers took DES during their first three months of pregnancy. Because DES taken early in pregnancy blocks the growth of normal genital tissue, DES daughters as young as seven were forced to undergo regular vaginal biopsies in an effort to find and remove these defects before they became lethal. In response to the suffering caused by these abnormalities, mothers and daughters exposed to DES banded together for mutual support, advice, and action. The first DES action group was formed on Long

Island, New York—a hotbed of DES prescribing. Ironically, the Long Island Breast Cancer Study Project ignored estrogen's role in increased breast cancer rates. Thanks to the efforts of Long Island DES activists in 1971, Peter Greenwald of the New York State Health Department collected information for a landmark report on the effects of DES.

While the DES task force was considering the harm caused to DES mothers and their daughters, it became clear that women were not alone in their anguish. We learned of a study of the relatively rare cancer of the testes in young men. Dr. Brian Henderson at the University of Southern California compared medical histories on 131 men under age forty who developed testicular cancer, with those who were cancer free. The researchers asked about a slew of possible risk factors including cigarette smoking, childhood illnesses such as mumps, and surgical history, including hernia repairs, and found that none of these explained why so many young men had developed this unusual cancer of the male reproductive system. Only one factor stood out—the mothers of these young men who contracted cancer of the testes had taken extra hormones during the seventh week of their pregnancies.

The dangers of synthetic estrogens are not limited to the women who have taken them, nor to their male or female children. Perhaps even more disconcerting is the growing evidence that such hormones pollute our soil and water and have a cascade of effects on wildlife. The hormone analogues used commercially are specifically designed to resist stomach acid "degradation" in order to remain effective. It was this very technology, the gastric durability developed in 1938 by Sir Charles Dodds, that ushered in the hormone age. Unfortunately, this same gastric durability allows chemicals to pass out of the body in our wastes, into our water and soil. Some three million women who live near the Thames River in London currently take birth control pills. Residues from 900 million contraceptive pills a year now pass into sewage systems and are released into surface or ground water nearby. Scientists believe this may explain the increasing incidence of hermaphroditic fish being caught in the Thames (at rates of up to 40 percent where urban sewage flows into the river).

Of even greater public health concern are the vast amounts of hormones fed to and excreted by livestock in this country. As I reported in my book *Women and the Crisis in Sex Hormones*, DES and other gastric-resistant hormones have been widely used in the livestock industry for more than half a century, from the 1940s through today. In sheer tonnage, the amounts of estrogen excreted by livestock and presumably seeping into our soil and water vastly exceed the amounts excreted by women taking physician-ordered contraceptives, fertility hormones, and menopause treatments.

Since the end of World War II, farmers had doled out massive amounts of DES and other synthetic estrogen to poultry, pigs, sheep, and cattle. Feed stores were selling it by the truckload, scrambling to meet a veterinary demand that was far greater than the human one. At the time my book was published in 1977, up to 85 percent of American livestock was being raised on DES. Though DES supporters claimed the hormone was administered to animals at "safe levels," a number of health experts insisted otherwise. They pointed out that DES was an established carcinogen. They noted that the 1958 Delaney Amendment to the Food, Drug and Cosmetic Law stipulated that "no [food] additive shall be deemed safe if it is found to induce cancer when injected by man or animal." While the law was later changed, it if had been enforced at the time it should have prevented DES from being so widely used.

Experts also noted that DES did little to improve the quality of meat. Some compared the fattening of animals with DES to certain practices that were a hanging offense in years gone by: The old-time farmer knew not to slaughter a female animal "in heat" because of the excess salt and water in tissues at the time. But some unscrupulous farmers gave their cows salt, followed by water, just before taking them to market. The stockyard operators soon learned to wait a couple of days until the cattle had excreted the salt and water before weighing the animals and paying for them. This process of salting and watering the stock, if discovered, was a crime, punishable by hanging in some areas of the country.

In the 1970s, DES was far from the only additive used to fatten up livestock. Nine other hormones were also in the mix. Many, like DES, had been banned from agriculture in other nations. These culprits included: chlormadinone acetate, permitted in feed for beef heifers and beef cows for synchronization of estrus (heat); progesterone, permitted for subcutaneous implantation in lambs and steers for growth promotion and feed efficiency; dienestrol diacetate, permitted in feed for broilers, fryers, and roasting chickens for the promotion of fat distribution and for tenderness and bloom; estradiol benzoate, used in combination with progesterone and testosterone; estradiol monopalmitate, permitted for injection under skin at the base of the skull of roasting chickens to produce more uniform fat distribution and improve finish; testosterone, permitted for subcutaneous ear injection in beef cattle to stimulate growth; testosterone proprionate, permitted for subcutaneous ear implantation in heifers to promote growth and increase feed efficiency; medroxyprogesterone acetate, permitted in feed for breeding cattle and ewes for the synchronization of estrus and ovulation; and melengestrol acetate, permitted in feed for heifers for growth stimulation, improved feed utilization, and suppression of estrus. Since DES was the additive known to have the most harmful effects, it was the one on which health advocates focused their ire. At my urging, the National Task Force on DES recommended that the use of DES in animal feed be banned. With a nod from Dr. Lester Crawford of the Veterinary

Bureau, the FDA withdrew its prior approval of the use of DES in animal feed to become effective in the 1980s.

The victory proved to be a pyrrhic one. The ban was a farce for two reasons: because some ranchers and poultry farms continued to use DES illegally, and because many started using other, less-well known estrogens or other growth stimulants in its place. Through the rest of the seventies — and through the eighties, nineties, and the dawn of the new millennium — I watched in horror as the use of estrogen and other hormones in livestock feed continued unabated. Today, many of the nine substances listed above are not only still in use but are being administered in major quantities. Today, farmers still commit the hanging offense of using hormones to pack livestock full of salt and water. In the year 2003, our meat may be steeped in even more hormones than it was when DES was banned in 1979. This reality greeted reporter Michael Pollan when he investigated the American cattle industry for a lengthy article that ran in the *New York Times Magazine* in March 2002. Pollan stared in awe as bleating calves were "funneled into a chute, herded along by a ranch hand yielding an electric prod, then clutched in a restrainer just long enough for another hand to inject a slow-release pellet of Reviar, a synthetic estrogen, in the back of the ear." Pollan learned that U.S. farmers raise an estimated 36 million beef cattle — and give hormones to roughly two-thirds of these animals. Estrogen advocates told Pollan that hormones "get a beef calf from 80 to 1,200 pounds in the span of just fourteen months" and can boost an animal's growth by 20 percent. They justified using estrogen because it seemed cost-effective. A hormone implant costing $1.50, they said, could add 50 pounds to the weight of a steer and yield a return of at least $25.

However, on the downside, Pollan noted that hormone-laced feed can change the pH level of a steer's digestive tract from basic to acidic — one reason 13 percent of feedlot cattle have abscessed livers by the time they are slaughtered. And, he reported measurable amounts of agricultural hormones can now be found in our meat, and that these hormones "contribute to the build-up of estrogenic compounds in our environment, which some scientists believe may explain falling sperm counts and premature maturation in girls."

Pollan noted that "recent studies have found elevated levels of synthetic hormones in feedlot waters; these persistent chemicals eventually wind up in the waterways downstream of feedlots, where scientists have found fish exhibiting abnormal sex characteristics." Indeed, reports of gender-bending aquatic animals are multiplying like minnows. When scientists from Britain's Environmental Agency examined fish in ten major rivers they found intersex males in every single one. Just under 50 percent of males had developed either eggs in their testes or female reproductive tracts. Researchers believed the main culprit was ethinyl estradiol, a synthetic estrogen used in the contraceptive pill. Dr. Charles Tyler of Exeter University, the lead researcher, said the hormone is "so exquisitely potent that some of the very concentrations where we are seeing effects on fish are below the detection limit that is presently in place for testing our drinking water."

Evidence of estrogenic effects also continues to surface in American waterways. For example, researchers from South Carolina's Clemson University discovered ponds affected by runoff from cattle farms contained male juvenile sunfish making the egg yolk protein normally produced by adult females while scientists in New Hampshire found frogs with elevated levels of estrogen—and deformed reproductive organs. In 2001, other researchers caught "female" fish in the Columbia River in Washington State. When they analyzed the genes of these fish, they discovered the "females" were actually males.

The most damning proof of estrogen pollution came in the summer of 2002, when the U.S. Geological Survey completed the first comprehensive study of chemical contaminants in our water. Researchers examined 139 streams and rivers in thirty states and found that 40 percent of waterways showed traces of estrogen or other reproductive hormones. When the results of the two-year survey were published, USGS scientist Herbert Burton noted that compounds with hormone-like properties "can affect the growth and development of aquatic life." Much of this pollution can be traced straight back to animal and human waste. When Andreas Daxenburger of the Technical University of Munich studied U.S. feedlots he discovered that animals shed about 10 percent of their progestin feed additive in their feces alone.

At the University of Florida researcher Louis J. Guillette, Jr. (who spent years studying undersized penises and other sexual abnormalities in Florida alligators linked to hormone exposure) tried to compare the runoff from feedlots that use hormones to the runoff from those that did not. The experiment failed because Guillette couldn't find a single cattle farm that didn't give growth-stimulating hormones to its livestock.

While not a single country has dealt with the issue of pharmaceutical or agricultural hormone contamination of water and soil, at least some of the world has paid attention to the problem of hormones found in livestock. The European Union, for instance, has banned the importation of hormone-treated meat since 1988. When synthetic hormones do surface, authorities officially act to put safety measures in place as noted. In July 2002, Provera (medroxyprogesterone acetate, a synthetic estrogen used in Prempro) was discovered in pig feed sent to farms in fifteen European countries. The culprit was water waste from an Irish processing plant owned by U.S. drug maker Wyeth-Ayerst. When authorities learned that the grain was tainted, they forced thousands of farmers to halt production and carefully weeded out the contaminated feed. Health advocates made certain that meat consumers were not exposed to hormones—a precaution that is foreign to the United States.

Just as we've shrugged off the problem of hormones in agriculture, we've ignored unsettling proof of what these hormones are doing to our environment. In the words of researcher Christian Daughter (who heads the environmental chemistry branch of the EPA's National Exposures Laboratory in Las Vegas, Nevada), "the United States is a late bloomer on the issue of these emerging organic wastewater contaminants, particularly pharmaceuticals."

So potent are some synthetic hormones that farm and veterinary-supply workers, scientists who handle but do not ingest hormone products, and others who are in an environment containing estrogen dust appear to be at an increased risk of cancer. In February 1982, Rutgers University in New Jersey was forced to close Smith Hall, its largest classroom building and home to the Institute of Animal Behavior, where experiments involving estrogen had been conducted. The buildings proved to be so heavily laced with growth-stimulating residues that work had to be halted. The Occupational Safety and Health Administration determined that the estrogen levels found in several areas of the building were so high they markedly increased the risk of cancer for those working in the area.

From the moment synthetic estrogens were first created, scientists have realized that these powerful agents could prove hazardous. We've known about hormones' adverse effects since the 1930s and 1940s, when estrogens were found to induce miscarriage, breast cancer, and blood clots in lab animals. For several decades, we've known about prepubescent girls, male lab workers, and male restaurant employees who all sprouted breasts after direct exposure to estrogen. Despite this evidence, the effects of the veterinary and pharmaceutical estrogens that animals and humans are being fed and excreting into the environment remain largely unmonitored and unchecked.

The Long Island Breast Cancer Research Project was particularly disappointing because Long Island itself presented a rich source for a serious study of the links between manufactured hormones and hormone-dependent cancers of the breast, uterus, ovaries, and testes. Nassau and Suffolk Counties, which were among the fastest-growing and most affluent communities in the United States in the 1940s, 1950s, and 1960s, attracted scores of cutting-edge obstetricians and gynecologists from the nation's most elite medical schools. Many of these physicians, enamored of the notion that they could exercise godlike powers over women's reproductive systems with synthetic hormones, prescribed estrogen-based drugs to thousands of Long Island women for everything from regulating menstrual periods to clearing up acne, preventing miscarriages, drying up leaky breasts, and promoting "feminine forever" youth.

In addition to these profligate medical uses of hormones, thousands of other men, women, and children may have been exposed to hormones on the farms that once dotted the Long Island landscape. Farm wives and their children, many of whom were responsible for feeding the chickens and other livestock, had handled DES-infused animal feed directly, boosting their chances of developing breast cancer or other hormonally tied cancer later in life. And untold tons of estrogen-laced farm animal and human wastes had seeped into the Long Island water and soil.

Yet, inexplicably, the Long Island study scientists focused on the possible link between breast cancer and a limited range of toxic chemical exposures, such as some pesticides or those found in toxic wastes. In truth, we have known for years that the women most likely to develop breast cancer were those who could pay for synthetic estrogen in the form of DES, the pill, or HRT. These affluent women were not likely to be living next door to sewage treatment plants and waste dumps, though they were more likely to have used pesticides inside their homes and in their gardens.

Reviewing the results of the Long Island study, I began to wonder if this was like the tobacco research I learned about years ago from two friends of mine in the public relations business, Ted Klein and Leonard Zahn. In the middle of the last century, the tobacco industry financed health studies of lung diseases. Specifically, in 1964, soon after the Surgeon General's report on smoking, the AMA accepted $15 million (the equivalent of near $100 million today) to fund tobacco-related research. In truth, some good work came from it. But their motive was not to foster solid research on heart or lung disease, but to divert attention from the primary role played by cigarettes in poor health. Perhaps the hormone industry played some behind-the-scenes role in the work of Long Island researchers. The protocols for both the Long Island breast cancer and the NIH endocrine disruptor studies make one wonder whether estrogen research is indeed objective and unbiased. Thanks to the machinations of American pharmaceutical companies (and thanks to smoke-and-mirrors studies by the scientists that they fund) we may never know the truth. Studies on environmental health are always hampered, in part because they are fundamentally complex. As cancer expert Devra Davis puts it in her National Book Award Finalist work, *When Smoke Ran Like Water*, "When all is said and done, the surprise is not how little we know about public health today, but how much we have been able to learn despite the barriers to science, the outright lying and deceptions and intimidation, and the political and economic pressures that continue to make it difficult to conduct studies at all."

While the Long Island and NIH studies were profoundly disappointing in their failure to ask about environmental and pharmaceutical hormones, there are some signs that U.S. authorities may be grudgingly waking up to the dangers of such contaminants. In May of 2002, Rep. Louise Slaughter (D-N.Y.) introduced legislation that would boost federal research on hormone disruptors by $500 million. The NIEHS's National Toxicology Program published its tenth report on carcinogens, including *all* steroidal estrogen products as confirmed causes of human cancer. Davis told me recently, "We know enough now to restrict our exposures to synthetic hormones. Of course, we need more research. We always need more research. But we also know that we should reduce our uses of many growth-stimulating compounds throughout the environment today."

While we wait, evidence keeps mounting that confirms the worries of scientists from past decades. In her book, Davis painstakingly documents troubling patterns of hormonally related cancer and other diseases. Why are more baby boys being born with smaller penises and undescended testes? Why are more young men developing testicular cancer throughout the industrial world? Why are deer and bear and whales and other wildlife showing up with deformities of their reproductive systems? Could this be related to the combined effects of hormones in the environment, from agricultural to pharmaceutical uses, to those agents found in toxic chemicals that can act like hormones when ingested, to undetected exposures to radiation, or to some combination of all of these?

Science remains incomplete on these matters, in part because the science is difficult. But, it is also true, as Davis and others make clear, that sometimes we know less than we should, because powerful forces have worked to make sure we remain uncertain.

Nobody can be sure whether environmental estrogens lie behind the quadrupling of infertility rates since 1965; if the sea of estrogens in which we live explains the fact that sperm counts are half of what they were in 1940; and if, like intersex fish and mutant frogs, male humans might begin to shed their broad shoulders and slowly morph into women. Faced with the possibility of an all-female planet, authorities might finally have to sidestep the pharmaceutical companies and take decisive action.

Appendix: Over the Menopausal Rainbow

With Toto in her arms, Dorothy rounds the fence post, runs into the house, and boards herself up in her bedroom as the tornado approaches. She's looked everywhere but can't find Auntie Em and or any of the farmhands. The tornado's force picks up and objects are blowing past her window. In the swirls of wind Dorothy sees the wicked witch fly by, vowing to get her, just before she is knocked unconscious.

The Wizard of Oz may just be a movie, but millions of women in the summer of 2002 were hit by a tornado just like Dorothy. The lives of 6 million American women on Prempro were turned upside down when the Women's Health Initiative announced it was halting a study of Prempro because the drug was shown to increase the risk of stroke, heart disease, and breast cancer in postmenopausal women. Add that to the revised guidelines for administering Premarin, the most widely prescribed hormone in the world, and what woman would not shut herself in her bedroom waiting for the storm to subside? How many women felt alone, not knowing what to do as the tornado of menopause, which is how the pharmaceutical companies would like you to view it, loomed in the distance?

Women today become overwhelmed, like Dorothy, questioning their hormone replacement options, feeling confused as options sail past the window. And like Dorothy, just as the maelstrom's full force hits, the only thing you can see are the pharmaceutical companies and their new drugs right outside your window; you're almost relieved to pass out on your bed and wake up in Oz.

We're Not in Kansas Anymore: Your Body Enters Menopause

Most women reach natural menopause between the ages of forty-five and fifty-five. Menopause represents the end of fertility in a woman's life and is the point at which menstruation ends. Natural menopause results from the decreased production of estrogen and progesterone by the ovaries as a woman ages. In contrast, surgical (or induced) menopause can cause a sudden loss of ovarian estrogen and the immediate initiation of menopause. Unlike natural menopause, during which estrogen levels drop gradually, when a woman undergoes surgical menopause, her symptoms, such as hot flashes, night sweats, and vaginal dryness, can be sudden and severe. Before we discuss the options available to women to treat their menopausal symptoms, it is important to understand the hormonal changes brought upon by menopause.

Except when menopause results from surgery, it is usually a gradual process beginning with fluctuations in the menstrual cycle. The menstrual cycle begins on the first day of menstrual flow (the menstrual phase, days 1 to 5). This shedding of the endometrial lining is the result of declining estrogen and progesterone toward the end of the previous cycle's phase. These low hormone levels stimulate the hypothalamus to produce gonadotropin-releasing hormone, which causes the pituitary gland to create and secrete follicle-stimulating hormone (FSH) and luteinizing hormone (LH).

FSH stimulates the growth of follicles in the ovary, one of which will produce a mature egg. LH stimulates estrogen secretion by the follicles. The follicles' secretion of estrogen begins a phase in which the levels of estrogen increase and the endometrium thickens in preparation for an egg (the proliferative phase, days 5 to 13). The proliferative phase ends with ovulation, when the follicle releases a mature egg. The last phase (the secretory phase, days 14 to 28) begins when the empty follicle becomes the corpus luteum, which secretes both progesterone and estrogen to thicken the endometrium in preparation for a fertilized egg. If fertilization does not occur, the estrogen and progesterone produced by the corpus luteum start to inhibit the production of LH and FSH. When the levels of LH drop, the corpus luteum begins to atrophy and stops producing estrogen and progesterone. The thickening of the endometrium can no longer be maintained and is shed as menstrual flow.

Typically, some time after a woman reaches the age of forty, estrogen production begins to lessen. The pituitary gland responds by secreting more FSH to spur on the ovaries. (This is why a key clinical sign that a woman is undergoing menopause is the presence of elevated levels of FSH in the blood and urine.) Ovulation is now sporadic, and even if FSH stimulates the ovaries to produce enough estrogen to prepare the endometrium for the first half of the menstrual cycle, without ovulation no progesterone is produced for the second half. The endometrium is built up to receive an egg yet does not mature enough to shed when no egg is implanted. As a result, the cycle is thrown off and bleeding can be delayed, or may go on longer than the normal five to seven days. Eventually the ovaries almost cease producing estrogen and menopause occurs. Contrary to the popular description of ovaries dying and postmenopausal women having no estrogen, women continue to produce upward of 10 percent of their former estrogen after menopause and throughout the rest of their lives.

Estrogen is not one hormone, but the name of a group of hormones. There are three principal forms of estrogen found in the human body: estrone, estradiol, and estriol. Estradiol is the primary estrogen produced by the ovaries. Estrone is formed from estradiol; it is a weak estrogen and is the most abundant estrogen found in the body after menopause. Estriol is produced in large amounts during pregnancy and is a product of the breakdown of estradiol. Before menopause, estradiol is the predominant estrogen. After menopause, estradiol levels drop more than estrone levels, so that estrone is the predominant estrogen. While estrogen gets all the attention, progesterone is just as essential to our body. It is synthesized in the body from cholesterol—as are all steroid hormones—and is influential in the second half of the menstrual cycle, as discussed above. Progesterone is a precursor to other hormones and can create and help to balance estrogen, testosterone, and cortisol, the stress hormone. Recently, testosterone has been receiving more attention for the role it plays in menopause. Testosterone is made in the ovaries and the adrenal glands, and it is influential in making many tissues, contributing to strength, energy, and sexual arousal.

When we left Dorothy she was unconscious on her bed as the tornado uprooted her house and the wind carried it over the rainbow. Dorothy wakes up in a strange place called Munchkin Land. But in our version of Munchkin Land, Dorothy is greeted not only by Glinda, the good witch, but also by hot flashes and insomnia, common menopausal occurrences called vasomotor symptoms.

Hot flashes are the most prominent symptom, which are experienced as an intense buildup in body heat, often followed by sweating and chills. The hot flash is still not fully understood; it is believed that diminished estrogen levels are somehow responsible. Withdrawal of estrogen causes an increase in the levels of the hormones FSH and LH. The higher the levels of FSH and LH, the more the blood vessels dilate, or enlarge, which increases blood flow to the skin, raising its temperature. Almost two-thirds of postmenopausal women have hot flashes, and 10 to 20 percent of all postmenopausal women find them nearly intolerable. The U.S. Bureau of the Census estimated that in 2001, almost 43 million women would be over fifty. Thus over 25 million women in the United States might have had hot flashes, and up to 4 million might have reported severe symptoms.

Vaginal atrophy—a thinning, drying, and loss of elasticity—can also occur when estrogen levels decline. Secondary results of vaginal atrophy are painful intercourse and a greater susceptibility to vaginal and urinary infections. Many women may not experience vaginal atrophy until years past menopause.

Some women report an accompanying increase in anxiety. Insomnia is also common; it may be caused by hot flashes or may be an independent symptom of hormonal changes. Mood changes also occur; their cause is likely to be a combination of sleeplessness, hormonal swings, and psychological factors as a woman undergoes this phase in her life.

After Dorothy is introduced to menopausal Munchkin Land, she desperately asks Glinda how she can return to Kansas, a place where her hormones are not out of control. Before Glinda can answer, the Wicked Witch of the West arrives to claim the ruby slippers—which are still on the feet of the witch crushed by Dorothy's house landing. Glinda quickly transfers the shoes onto Dorothy's feet. The wicked witch claims the slippers will work only for her and are of no use to Dorothy, but Glinda tells Dorothy the slippers must be very powerful if the witch wants them so badly and that Dorothy should never take them off. In a huff of smoke the wicked witch takes off, vowing to get Dorothy and her little dog, too. We don't know the power of the ruby slippers yet, but Glinda tells Dorothy the slippers will protect her on her journey to see the wizard, the only person who may be able to help her get home.

This all-powerful Wizard of Oz is Dorothy's only hope. Sound familiar? Women in general made an average of 4.6 doctor visits in 2001 and have made hormone replacement therapy a $2.75 billion industry to date. How does it happen that a natural occurrence in life drives us to the doctor's office in such numbers? Or is it that menopause has been taken away from us and turned into something else—something we believe is beyond our control and something only a doctor has the answers to? Menopause has been medicalized: Medicalization is a process whereby more and more of everyday life comes under medical influence and supervision so that medical definitions and treatments emerge for previously nonmedical problems. Childbirth is a classic example of a natural event that is now medically managed.

The process by which the medical industry has medicalized menopause allows them to gain what is called social control. Social control allows doctors to lay claim to all activities concerning a medicalized condition. An ever more devastating outgrowth of social control is the phenomenon of the sick role. If the medical industry can control any situation and make something medical just by defining it as such, then they can also decide who is healthy and who is ill. Doctors and pharmaceutical companies profit by placing women in the sick role and making them feel as though they have a disease only the medical industry can fix. Like Dorothy, many women fall under the spell of social control and believe only the wizard, doctor, or pharmaceutical company can help them.

To start her journey Dorothy is told to follow the yellow brick road. Of course, we know the road for menopausal treatment is more like a street lined with gold leading up to the door of the pharmaceutical companies. The drug industry has quite a number of elaborate ways to make you buy their products. One method is to enlist the help of doctors in boosting their product. The pharmaceutical companies accomplish this by spending $8,000 to $13,000 per physician annually in gifts to physicians such as lunches, books, and stethoscopes; free attendance at conferences; and all-expenses-paid trips to meetings. These methods pay off when you realize that only 27 percent of physicians prescribe generic options for their patients; this means the other 83 percent are pushing higher-priced brand-name drugs. Another way the drug industry gets you is through direct-to-consumer advertising; in 1999 the pharmaceutical industry spent more than $1.8 billion to get your attention. Again, this seems to work; a study by *Prevention* magazine found that a third of consumers who had seen direct-to-consumer advertisements went on to speak with their health care providers about the medicine advertised. The proven track record for these methods allowed Wyeth to increase the price of Premarin by a staggering 18 percent in 2001 alone, which far outpaced the U.S. cost of living increase of only 3 percent in 2001.

THE OPTIONS: A JOURNEY TO OZ

As Dorothy and Toto travel down the yellow brick road they come to their first fork in the road. Luckily, there is a scarecrow pointing the way to Oz. But when Dorothy looks again, she sees the scarecrow has changed the direction he is pointing. Dorothy gets confused and asks the scarecrow which is the right way, but he admits that he doesn't really know the way to Oz. This lack of clear direction might seem familiar in light of the Women's Health Initiative revelation. It almost seems every time a claim is made by a drug company, a study comes out the next day to refute it.

Over the last fifty years, the thrust of estrogen treatment has been to alleviate the symptoms of menopause, but the pharmaceutical companies have pushed women to think of HRT as long-term health maintenance. The findings of the Women's Health Initiative study are forcing the pharmaceutical industry to backpedal on the notion that a woman should take estrogen for the remainder of her life after menopause. In fact, Wyeth, the manufacturer of Premphase, Premarin, and Prempro, recommends women stay on these drugs for only the shortest amount of time possible. It should be noted that new recommendations and guidelines are released almost daily by the FDA, prescription drug watchdog groups, or pharmaceutical companies themselves.

Many women still feel compelled to find a treatment for symptoms of menopause, and it has become necessary to rethink what constitutes the ideal estrogen. Following is a description of some of the options available to women today. This is not an endorsement of any kind of therapy, just a guide to assist you in better understanding your options.

Progestins

Dorothy and Toto, now joined by the Scarecrow, find an abandoned home and start looking around the property; they find a tin man rusted through and frozen in position while chopping wood. The Tin Man appears to be trying to tell them something. They realize he is asking them to find his oil can and lubricate his joints. Once the oil is applied everywhere, the Tin Man explains that he had been chopping wood one day when it began to rain; he couldn't reach his oil can and eventually rusted through. We learn from the Tin Man that missing one small ingredient can have dire consequences. For many women, progestins are the oil can for their bodies. Without progestins to balance the hormonal cycle, estrogen overstimulates the tissue lining the uterus and causes uncontrolled growth, a condition known as hyperplasia. Hyperplasia, if atypical and untreated, may develop into uterine cancer. While much of the emphasis is on estrogen replacement, it is crucial to remember the important role of progestins.

Progestins are recommended for women with a uterus who are on estrogen therapy to counteract the effects of estrogen on the uterine lining. Doctors commonly prescribe a combination of estrogen and progesterone therapy for menopausal women who still have a uterus to help alleviate vasomotor symptoms such as hot flashes while still protecting the endometrium.

Ironically, after a year, less than 40 percent of women who started hormone treatment continue to take their medications. The main reasons women discontinue hormone treatment are bleeding and breast tenderness. Bleeding is exactly what should happen when a progestin is added. Your body is shedding the lining of the uterus and is decreasing the chance that endometrial cancer will develop.

There are two types of progestins: natural progestins, also called progesterone, and synthetic progestins. Most people assume that a synthetic hormone is made in a lab, whereas the natural hormone originates directly from nature. This is not the case. Both are made in the lab, and even synthetics can be concocted from natural products. The difference between the two is not their source—whether they come from soy or yam or are developed in a test tube. The distinction lies in their basic molecular arrangement. If the chemical structure of the product identically matches that of a woman's naturally occurring hormone, it is considered to be natural. Simply, a natural hormone is intended to mimic the human female hormone. The natural form of progesterone appears to have several benefits. The bioidentical version helps to balance estrogen as well as other sex hormones; it is utilized more efficiently and leaves the body quickly, as do our own hormones.

Women may be less aware of the option to take natural hormones because they have not been subjected to the extensive research of the synthetic hormones. Pharmaceutical companies have little incentive to spend millions of dollars to research and manufacture a product they can't exclusively patent, as is the case with natural hormones. However, the device that delivers the hormone, such as a patch or an applicator tube for a cream, can be patented, which is why some pharmaceutical companies market bioidentical hormones. Synthetic hormones, on the other hand, are made by altering the molecular structure of a hormone enough so that it can be patented. But natural estrogen and progesterone are available and FDA-approved, just like the synthetics, and can be prescribed by your doctor.

Examples of Available Progesterones

Prometrium is a natural form of finely ground progesterone made from wild yams, known as micronized progesterone. Micronized means it has been broken down into little particles to enable your body to metabolize it more easily. Before this process was discovered, many women couldn't take natural progesterone orally because it was absorbed badly and became inactive when swallowed.

Prometrium is used to induce the natural shedding of the lining of the uterus and thus prevent overgrowth of the endometrium of postmenopausal women who have not had a hysterectomy and are receiving estrogen replacement therapy. The suggested dose for Prometrium capsules is 200 mg capsules taken orally once a day, for 12 sequential days per

28-day cycle for cyclical therapy and 100 to 200 mg daily for continuous therapy. Prometrium is usually taken orally, but it can also be used as a vaginal suppository. In the latter case, the capsule is inserted directly in the vagina.

A note of warning: Do not take the Prometrium brand of progesterone if you are allergic or sensitive to peanuts. Prometrium capsules contain peanut oil and should never be used by people allergic to peanuts.

Crinone is a progesterone vaginal gel designed to deliver progesterone directly to the part of the body where it is needed. Crinone is used to treat the absence of menstruation due to progesterone deficiency. Like Prometrium, Crinone causes the uterus to shed its lining as it would during normal menstruation. The suggested dosage is every other day for 12 days of the month for cyclical therapy or twice a week for continuous therapy. Applied to the vagina, the gel adheres to the walls of the vagina so that the progesterone can be absorbed locally, with minimal absorption by the bloodstream. The supposed benefit of this method is that because the progesterone goes directly from the vagina to the target organ, the uterus, you don't get high blood levels of progesterone, which means that you may get the benefits of progesterone with few side effects.

A note of warning: In 2000, Crinone was voluntarily recalled from the marketplace due to a problem with the dispenser of the gel. For more information on its availability, speak with your doctor or pharmacist or contact the manufacturer. Do not use Crinone at the same time as other vaginal products. If you are using another vaginal product, use it at least six hours before or after a dose of topical progesterone unless specifically directed to do otherwise by your doctor.

Do not take progesterone without first talking to your doctor if you have a bleeding or blood-clotting disorder, breast cancer, cancer of a genital organ, liver disease, or undiagnosed vaginal bleeding.

Before taking this medication, tell your doctor if you have epilepsy or a seizure disorder, migraines, asthma, kidney disease, heart disease, diabetes, or a history of depression.

Possible serious side effects of progesterone are an allergic reaction (difficulty breathing; closing of your throat; swelling of your lips, tongue, or face; or hives); shortness of breath or pain in your chest; a sudden severe headache; visual changes; a painful, red, swollen leg; numbness or tingling in an arm or leg; prolonged heavy vaginal bleeding; stomach or side pain; or yellowing of your skin or eyes.

Other side effects may be more likely to occur, such as dizziness; drowsiness; headache; breast pain or tenderness; abdominal pain or distension; diarrhea; vaginal discharge; or mood changes, anxiety, and irritability.

Examples of Available Progestins

Amen, Curretab, Cycrin, and Provera are all brand-name oral progestins with the main active ingredient of medroxyprogesterone (MPA). MPA is in effect the conjugated estrogen of the progesterone world. MPA is the most commonly prescribed progestin and has been used in the most HRT studies. This synthetic form of progesterone is called a C21 progestin and is made by adding chemical groups to progesterone. But MPA often causes PMS-like side effects in many women—sometimes to such a degree that women want to stop HRT completely. In addition, MPA may detract from some of the heart-health aspects of estrogen. So it's usually recommended that you take the smallest amount that will protect against endometrial buildup.

Medroxyprogesterone is used to treat conditions such as irregular or abnormal uterine bleeding and lack of menstruation. The suggested dosage for Provera is 2.5 mg daily for continuous therapy or 5 to 10 mg a day for 10 to 12 days beginning on the 13th or 15th day of your cycle for cyclic therapy. The suggested dosage for Amen, Curretab, and Cycrin are 2.5 mg daily for continuous therapy or 5 to 10 mg daily for 5 to 10 days beginning on the 16th day of your cycle.

A note of warning: A report issued by the National Cancer Institute found women who used HRT sustained a greater risk of developing breast cancer. This is because commonly used progestins, like Provera, have androgenic activity, which can stimulate breast cells. Also, while taking medroxyprogesterone avoid smoking (smoking greatly increases the risk of blood clot formation); excessive salt intake (too much salt may cause fluid retention and discomfort); and prolonged exposure to sunlight.

Do not take medroxyprogesterone without the approval of your doctor if you have a bleeding or blood-clotting disorder, any type of breast or uterine cancer, or liver or gallbladder disease. Before taking this medication, tell your doctor if you have epilepsy or a seizure disorder, migraines, asthma, kidney disease, heart disease, or diabetes.

Possible serious side effects of medroxyprogesterone are an allergic reaction (difficulty breathing; closing of your throat; swelling of your lips, tongue, or face; or hives); shortness of breath or pain in your chest; a sudden severe headache; visual changes; a painful, red, swollen leg; numbness or tingling in an arm or leg; prolonged heavy vaginal bleeding; stomach or side pain; yellowing of your skin or eyes.

Other side effects may be more likely to occur, such as changes in appetite or weight, swelling of your hands or feet, changes in your menstrual cycle, depression, acne, an increase in body or facial hair or hair loss, tenderness of the breasts, nausea, headache or insomnia, changes in your voice, or areas of darker skin.

Before taking medroxyprogesterone, tell your doctor if you are taking any of the following medications: insulin or an oral diabetes medicine such as glipizide (Glucotrol), glyburide (DiaBeta, Micronase, Glynase), chlorpropamide (Diabinese), tolazamide (Tolinase), and tolbutamide (Orinase); bromocriptine (Parlodel); aminoglutethimide (Cytadren); phenobarbital (Solfoton, Luminal); or chlorpromazine (Thorazine), fluphenazine (Prolixin), mesoridazine (Serentil), perphenazine (Trilafon), prochlorperazine (Compazine), promazine (Sparine), thioridazine (Mellaril), or trifluoperazine (Stelazine).

Aygestin and Norlutate are brand-name oral progestins with the main active ingredient norethindrone acetate. Another synthetic progesterone, norethindrone acetate (NTA), is a C19 progestin, made from testosterone. Different chemical groups are added and subtracted, eliminating the male properties from the hormone and forming an absorbable, stable progestin. It is stronger than MPA, so you need smaller dosages.

Norethindrone acetate is commonly prescribed to women who have had problems dealing with side effects from Provera or Cycrin, and is said to help reduce the breast tenderness and bloating that are often caused by MPA. Suggested dosage for Aygestin is 2.5 to 10 mg for 5 to 10 days. Suggested dosage for Norlutate is 2.5 to 10 mg from the 5th through 25th day of your cycle.

A note of warning: Progestin withdrawal bleeding usually occurs within three to seven days after discontinuing Aygestin therapy.

Do not take norethindrone without the approval of your doctor if you have a history of blood clots in the legs, lungs, eyes, brain, or elsewhere; liver impairment or disease; known or suspected cancer of the breast; undiagnosed vaginal bleeding; hypersensitivity to Aygestin tablets.

Possible side effects of taking norethindrone are breakthrough bleeding, spotting, change in menstrual flow, edema, changes in weight, changes in cervical secretions, jaundice, rashes, mental depression, acne, breast enlargement/tenderness, headache/migraine, abnormalities of liver tests, mood swings, nausea, insomnia, changes in libido, hirsutism, or loss of scalp hair.

Micronor, known as the mini-pill, is a synthetic norethindrone-based progestin similar to Aygestin, but it has another chemical group attached to it. It's widely used as a progesterone-only birth control pill, one that has fewer risks because it doesn't contain estrogen. But it's also used in hormone supplements as a progesterone replacement. It's a very low dose progestin—only .35 mg daily. Because it's such a low dose, it's most commonly prescribed in continuous HRT—you take both estrogen and Micronor every day. Many women claim success with Micronor because, for some women, it stops breakthrough bleeding (bleeding while on continuous HRT) quickly, usually within 9 months.

Is Estrogen Still the King of the Forest?

Now we find Dorothy, Toto, the Scarecrow, and the Tin Man entering a dark forest, where they become frightened of the possibilities of lions, tigers, and bears. Suddenly a lion jumps onto the path in front of them and tries to scare them, telling them that he is king of the forest. Of course we learn he's a cowardly lion who only dreams of being king of the forest. But the lion's hype and bravado were convincing enough for a time, like the manufacturer of Prempro and Premarin. After the announcement by the Women's Health Initiative, women began to wonder if there was any evidence to the claims and hype of these drugs. It left us wondering: Is estrogen treatment still the king of the forest?

Again, estrogen is not one hormone, it is the name of a group of hormones. There are three principal forms of estrogen found in the human body: estrone, estradiol, and estriol. Estradiol is produced by the ovaries each month and is the estrogen most constant in our body throughout life. Estrone is the estrogen associated with the menopausal woman; it is made in the adrenal glands and the ovaries and is derived from body fat. Estriol is produced in the ovaries and the placenta during pregnancy and is the weakest of the three estrogens. Like progestins, estrogen therapy falls under many different subheadings.

Many pills, patches, and injectibles are based on only one human estrogen rather than a mix of the three estrogen compounds. While some of these hormones may be natural in the sense that they are similar to the hormones found in our bodies, limiting your hormone replacement to one type of estrogen could create an overall hormonal imbalance, since the principal blueprint for estrogen in the human female body is based on three compounds, not one.

Remember that unopposed estrogen increases risk for uterine cancer, so it is recommended only for women who have had a hysterectomy. Without progesterone to balance the hormonal cycle, estrogen overstimulates the tissue lining the uterus and causes uncontrolled growth, a condition known as hyperplasia. Hyperplasia, if atypical and untreated, may develop into uterine cancer. Any woman with an intact uterus who is taking unopposed estrogen therapy should have annual endometrial biopsies and report any vaginal bleeding immediately. Please note that this warning applies to all of the estrogen options described below.

Conjugated Estrogens

Conjugated in the medical sense means a chemical compound that is formed by the joining of two or more compounds. Since Premarin is derived from the urine of many mares, it is a conjugated estrogen. It is also the biggest brand name of estrogen—in fact, it's long been in the top five best-selling drugs overall in the country—and it's the one that doctors often automatically prescribe when you say you're ready to go on HRT. On the U.S. market since 1942, Premarin is the form of estrogen used in the bulk of the research studies on HRT, which means that most things you read about estrogen are actually specifically about Premarin. Remember, since the halting of the WHI study, Wyeth, the manufacturer of Premarin, recommended that women who are taking Premarin stay on it for the shortest possible length of time.

When you take conjugated estrogens, your body converts them into active estrogens and uses them as it would the estrogen your ovaries have produced. Premarin is a mixture of over ten different estrogens—including estrone (which we make in our own bodies) and equilin and equilenin (horse estrogen, which of course we don't make in our own bodies). Because it comes from horse urine, the pharmaceutical company that makes Premarin (Wyeth Pharmaceuticals) considers it a natural estrogen. They are technically right; after all, horse urine is definitely natural. But by most standard definitions of natural as it applies to HRT, Premarin isn't considered one of the naturals, since it isn't identical to the estrogen we produce in our own bodies. Keep in mind the human female's reproductive system is quite different in makeup from a mare's. We use three estrogens in approximately the following ratios: estriol (60–90 percent), estrone (10–20 percent), and estradiol (10–20 percent). Premarin is a mixture of estrone (75–80 percent), equilin (6–5 percent), and estradiol, plus other horse estrogens (5–19 percent). The estrogen found in the greatest amount in the human female body, estriol, is completely left out and the proportion of estrone is far higher in Premarin than occurs in women naturally. And of course equilin and other horse estrogens are not included in a human's natural chemical makeup.

Premarin is used to treat moderate to severe hot flashes and night sweats associated with menopause and vaginal dryness. Suggested dosage: Premarin is available orally in 0.3, 0.625, 0.9, 1.25, and 2.5 mg doses. It is taken once daily for 25 days for cyclical therapy. And for continuous therapy it is taken once daily with a progestin.

Some doctors believe women suffer pronounced side effects from Premarin because it is so different from a woman's natural hormonal makeup. Also, Premarin is not metabolized in the body the same way as human hormones are. A woman's body contains all the essential enzymes and cofactors it needs to process its native hormones when they are present in their natural proportions. The more potent hormones like estradiol naturally break down into weaker compounds. However, Premarin doesn't contain the necessary enzymes and cofactors to metabolize equilin, and as a result that form of estrogen stays in the body, producing a more potent and long-lasting effect on our estrogen receptors. Levels of equilin metabolites (products of metabolism) can remain elevated in the body for up to 13 weeks or more after being ingested, due to storage and slow release from fat tissues.

Notes of warning: First, because of the potential risk of heart attack, stroke, breast cancer, and blood clots, use of Premarin should be limited to the shortest duration consistent with treatment goals and risks for the individual woman, and should be discussed with your physician. Second, it appears that you may get a higher amount of estrogen in your blood with Premarin than you do with some other estrogen products. The culprit here is the equilin. The amount of equilin you get from Premarin is much higher than your normal level of the human estrogens, estradiol and estrone. Because it is so strong, it appears to tax your liver more than other nonequine estrogens do, which can be a problem especially if you have a history of liver disease in your family or have had liver disease yourself; smoke; are obese; or have high blood pressure.

Do not take conjugated estrogens without first talking to your doctor if you have a circulation, bleeding, or blood-clotting disorder; undiagnosed abnormal vaginal bleeding; or any type of breast, uterine, or hormone-dependent cancer.

Before taking conjugated estrogens, tell your doctor if you have high blood pressure, angina, or heart disease; high levels of cholesterol or triglycerides in your blood; liver disease; kidney disease; asthma; epilepsy; migraines; diabetes; depression; gallbladder disease; uterine fibroids; or had a hysterectomy.

Possible serious side effects of conjugated estrogens include an allergic reaction (difficulty breathing, closing of your throat, swelling of your lips, tongue, or face, or hives); a blood clot (pain, redness, and swelling in an arm or leg, shortness of breath, chest pain, headache, blurred vision, or confusion); a lump in a breast; or liver damage (yellowing of the skin or eyes, nausea, abdominal pain or discomfort, unusual bleeding or bruising, severe fatigue).

Possible less serious side effects that may be more likely to occur are decreased appetite, nausea, or vomiting; swollen or tender breasts; acne or skin color changes; decreased sex drive; migraine headaches or dizziness; water retention (swollen hands, feet, or ankles); problems with wearing contact lenses; depression; or changes in your menstrual cycle or breakthrough bleeding.

Before taking conjugated estrogens, tell your doctor if you are taking any of the following medicines: an anticoagulant (blood thinner) such as warfarin (Coumadin); a thyroid medication such as Synthroid, Levoxyl, Levothroid, and others; insulin or an oral diabetes medicine such as glipizide (Glucotrol) or glyburide (DiaBeta, Micronase); tamoxifen (Nolvadex);

didanosine (Videx); phenytoin (Dilantin) or ethotoin (Peganone); carba-mazepine (Tegretol); phenobarbital (Solfoton, Luminal); primidone (Myso-line); or rifampin (Rifadin).

Premarin Vaginal Cream is also available to treat certain symptoms of menopause such as degeneration (thinning and shrinkage) of the vagina and vulvae. Standard dosage is 2 to 4 g cyclically to start.

A note of warning: Topical and vaginal conjugated estrogens may weaken some barrier forms of contraception such as latex condoms, diaphragms, and cervical caps. Talk to your doctor about adequate forms of birth control while using topical and vaginal conjugated estrogens if birth control is desired. Do not use any other vaginal medications without first talking to your doctor while using topical and vaginal conjugated estrogens.

Cenestin is a new synthetic form of conjugated plant estrogens from compounds found in yams and soy. In effect, then, it's the plant version of Premarin. It consists of nine different estrogens synthesized from plant sources. These estrogens include synthesized equine estrogens, so the pros and cons of Premarin apply here as well. On one hand, it's an option for women who like the idea of Premarin but are unhappy with the notion of horse urine. But as the estrogens are horse estrogens synthesized from plants, they're still not the same as human estrogens.

Cenestin is used for the treatment of menopausal symptoms like hot flashes. Standard dosage is 0.625, 0.9, and 1.25 mg oral tablet daily.

Examples of Estradiol-Based Estrogens

Estradiol is the estrogen our ovaries produce the most of during our reproductive years, so when you take estradiol as a hormone supplement, you are to some degree replacing the estrogen you used to make with its bioidentical twin. Taken orally, estradiol enters your gastrointestinal tract, is metabolized by your liver, and is converted into estrone—the estrogen your body has the most of after menopause

Estrace and Gynodiol are both estradiol-based oral tablets. They are bioidentical to natural estrogen and are made from plant sources that are micronized—broken down into little pieces—so the hormone is easily absorbed and used by your body.

Estrace and Gynodiol are used to treat vasomor symptoms and vaginal atrophy. Suggested dosage: Estrace is available in doses of 0.5, 1.0, and 2.0 mg daily. Gynodiol is available in 1 mg and 2 mg, which may be prescribed if the initial 1 mg dose fails to help eliminate symptom. Most recently, Gynodiol became available in a 1.5 mg dosage—since many women need something in between the 2 and the 1 mg levels.

Estradiol is most widely prescribed in the form of skin patches and creams and is gaining on Premarin in popularity. The Estraderm patch, a reservoir patch, was the first widely available estrogen patch and is still one of the most used today. Like the reservoir patches that were first designed, new patches continuously release natural, bioidentical estrogen into your system, but they tend to cause less skin irritation. The matrix patch was first introduced in 1995, when the Climara patch came out. A year later, the makers of the Estraderm patch came out with their version of a matrix patch, Vivelle. Next came Fempatch, a lower-dose estrogen patch. And most recently Vivelle came out with a new super-tiny patch—the Vivelle-Dot, about the size of a nickel or postage stamp. In all cases, the patch doesn't have the bubble that the Estraderm TTS patch does. Instead, it's a flat, translucent patch that lies flat under your clothes. In addition, the matrix delivery system appears to deliver estrogen more steadily, maintaining more stable blood levels of estrogen. But you get a slightly lower level of estrogen in your blood from the matrix patch than you do with the reservoir patch Estraderm TTS—about 70 picograms of estradiol from the .1

mg matrix patch as compared to 100 picograms from the corresponding Estraderm patch. Manufacturers tout as a benefit of the patch the fact that the hormone bypasses your liver while you get a steady, continuous dosage of estrogen into your system—bioidentical to human estradiol. Patches may be a better choice for smokers—as studies have indicated that oral estrogen may not deliver the same amount of estrogen to smokers as non-smokers, while patches don't appear to have this same problem.

Estraderm is a plant-derived estrogen patch. These are reservoir patches—transparent ovals with adhesive like a Band-Aid, and a fluid reservoir like a bubble in the middle. This bubble contains the estrogen, which is transmitted through your skin. You just apply it to unexposed skin—your buttocks, thighs, or lower abdomen—and forget about it until it's time to change it, which you do every $3^1/_2$ to 4 days. It usually takes less than 4 hours to reach the therapeutic level of estrogen in your system, and as with other patches, the estrogen is delivered continuously to your body.

Estraderm is used to treat vasomotor symptoms. It comes in both 50 mcg and 100 mcg dosages, with the 50 mcg patch being the most commonly prescribed initially.

Some women report skin irritation from the patch, which they attribute to the adhesive—especially in more sensitive areas, such as your lower abdomen. About 15 to 20 percent of the women using the Estraderm patch develop blotches and welts under and around the patch. You may be able to get around this, though, by moving the patch to less sensitive skin areas, such as the buttocks or thighs. In addition, using vitamin E or cortisone cream may help soothe the irritated skin. The second problem that a number of Estraderm users have reported: The edges often get rolled, less "stick-able," and generally messy. This isn't a huge problem, but it can get annoying—and sometimes embarrassing if the patch suddenly stops sticking at an inopportune moment.

Alora, Climara, Vivelle, Vivelle-Dot, and Fempatch are other patch options. They are all plant-derived estradiol and are sources of continuous estrogen. Most women report report better adhesion with these brands, and Vivelle and Alora's wide range of available dosages allows for more flexibility than other patches. The Vivelle-Dot's size is so small — the smallest available — that it's nearly undetectable, a real plus for people who are active and who don't want the hassle of the larger patches. Many women who suffer from migraine headaches claim they do better with an estrogen patch than with estrogen products in pill form.

Like Estraderm, these patches are used to treat many of the symptoms of perimenopause and menopause. They all come in a range of dosages, and some patches have to be changed twice a week, while others can stay on for a whole week at time. Climara is available in a range of 0.025, 0.05, 0.075, and 0.1 mg; Vivelle and Vivelle-Dot are available in ranges of 0.0375, 0.05, 0.075, and 0.1; Fempatch comes in a .025 mg dose; and Alora is available in doses of 0.05, 0.075, and 0.1 mg.

Esclim, just introduced in late 1999, is the newest estradiol patch available — but one with a key difference: It's stretchable, which makes it less prone to come off or come unstuck. As with other estrogen replacement therapies, the most commonly reported side effects typically include breast tenderness, headache, nausea, and abdominal pain. Esclim can be used by women who experience moderate to severe vasomotor symptoms associated with menopause. It also comes in a wide range of dosages available — from 0.025 up to 0.1, which may make it easier to find the best dosage for your specific needs. Standard dosage: 0.025, 0.0375, 0.05, 0.075, and 0.1 mg.

Estring is an elastomer ring containing 2 mg of estradiol, the major naturally occurring estrogen produced in the ovaries of fertile women. The Estring ring is inserted into the upper portion of the vagina, where it releases 50 to 60 percent of the estradiol, providing a consistent low-dose of estrogen for 3 months. Estring is used to treat local symptoms of vaginal atrophy. The ring should remain in place for 90 days. It should then be removed and replaced by a new ring, if prescribed by your doctor. If at any time the ring falls out, rinse it with warm water and reinsert it. If it slides down into the lower part of the vagina, use a finger to reinsert it. The ring does not need to be removed during sexual intercourse. It should not be felt by either partner. If it is bothersome, it can be removed, rinsed with warm water, and reinserted following intercourse.

Estrace Vaginal Cream is another form of estradiol from plants. Estradiol vaginal products release estrogen that is absorbed directly through the skin of the vaginal wall. Estrace Vaginal Cream is used to treat certain symptoms of menopause such as dryness, burning, and itching of the vaginal area and urgency or irritation with urination. Suggested dosage of the cream form is 2 to 4 mg a day for 1 to 2 weeks, then reduce the dose by half.

Do not use estradiol without first talking to your doctor if you have a circulation, bleeding, or blood-clotting disorder; undiagnosed abnormal vaginal bleeding; or any type of breast, uterine, or hormone-dependent cancer.

Before using estradiol, tell your doctor if you have high blood pressure, angina, or heart disease; high levels of cholesterol or triglycerides in your blood; liver disease; kidney disease; asthma; epilepsy; migraines; diabetes; depression; gallbladder disease; uterine fibroids; had a hysterectomy (uterus removed) ; a narrow, short, or prolapsed vagina; vaginal irritation; or a vaginal infection.

If you experience any of the following serious side effects of estradiol, stop using estradiol and seek emergency medical attention: an allergic reaction (difficulty breathing; closing of your throat; swelling of your lips, tongue, or face; or hives); shortness or breath or pain in your chest; a painful, red, swollen leg; abnormal vaginal bleeding; pain, swelling, or tenderness in the abdomen; severe headache or vomiting, dizziness, faintness or changes in vision or speech; yellowing of the skin or eyes; or a lump in a breast.

Other side effects may be more likely to occur, such as decreased appetite, nausea, or vomiting; swollen breasts; acne or skin color changes; decreased sex drive; migraine headaches or dizziness; vaginal pain, dryness, or discomfort; water retention (swollen hands, feet, or ankles); depression; or changes in your menstrual cycle or breakthrough bleeding.

Before using estradiol, tell your doctor if you are taking any of the following medicines: an anticoagulant (blood thinner) such as warfarin (Coumadin); or insulin or an oral diabetes medicine such as glipizide (Glucotrol) and glyburide (DiaBeta, Micronase); a thyroid medication such as Synthroid, Levoxyl, Levothroid, and others; tamoxifen (Nolvadex); didanosine (Videx); phenytoin (Dilantin) or ethotoin (Peganone); carbamazepine (Tegretol); phenobarbital (Solfoton, Luminal); primidone (Mysoline); or rifampin (Rifadin).

Examples of Estropipate-Based Estrogens

Another estrogen that is plant-derived, estropipate is made from purified crystalline estrone. In effect, then, when you take estropipate, you're getting the final by-product of estradiol and conjugated estrogens, since the liver converts the estrogens in them to estrone. Because it is weaker than the other estrogens, you need to take a higher dosage of estropipate to get the same levels of estradiol and estrone in your blood system you get from taking a standard dose of either conjugated estrogens or micronized estradiol. It's often prescribed to women who have side effects from the other estrogens, such as breast tenderness and bloating.

Ogen and Ortho-Est are estropipate estrogen replacement drugs. They are used for the treatment of moderate to severe vasomotor symptoms associated with the menopause and for treatment of vulval and vaginal atrophy.

Standard dosage for Ogen tablets ranges from one .625 tablet to two 2.5 tablets per day. Tablets should be taken in cycles of 3 weeks on and 1 week off according to your doctor's instructions.

Standard dosage for Ortho-Est Tablets ranges from half a tablet to 4 tablets per day of Ortho-Est 1.25 or 1 to 8 tablets of Ortho-Est .625. Tablets should be taken in cycles of 3 weeks on and 1 week off according to your doctor's instructions.

Do not take estropipate without first talking to your doctor if you have a circulation, bleeding, or blood-clotting disorder; undiagnosed abnormal vaginal bleeding; or any type of breast, uterine, or hormone-dependent cancer.

Before taking estropipate, tell your doctor if you have high blood pressure, angina, or heart disease; high levels of cholesterol or triglycerides in your blood; liver disease; kidney disease; asthma; epilepsy; migraines; diabetes; depression; gallbladder disease; uterine fibroids; or had a hysterectomy.

Possible side effects of estropipate include an allergic reaction (difficulty breathing; closing of your throat; swelling of your lips, tongue, or face, or hives); a blood clot (pain, redness, and swelling in an arm or leg, shortness of breath, chest pain, headache, blurred vision, or confusion); a lump in a breast; or liver damage (yellowing of the skin or eyes, nausea, abdominal pain or discomfort, unusual bleeding or bruising, severe fatigue).

Other side effects may be more likely to occur, such as decreased appetite, nausea, or vomiting; swollen or tender breasts; acne or skin color changes; decreased sex drive; migraine headaches or dizziness; water retention (swollen hands, feet, or ankles); problems with wearing contact lenses; depression; or changes in your menstrual cycle or breakthrough bleeding.

Before taking estropipate, tell your doctor if you are taking any of the following medicines: an anticoagulant (blood thinner) such as warfarin (Coumadin); a thyroid medication such as Synthroid, Levoxyl, Levothroid, and others; insulin or an oral diabetes medicine such as glipizide (Glucotrol) or glyburide (DiaBeta, Micronase); tamoxifen (Nolvadex); didanosine (Videx); phenytoin (Dilantin) or ethotoin (Peganone); carbamazepine (Tegretol); phenobarbital (Solfoton, Luminal); primidone (Mysoline); or rifampin (Rifadin).

Examples of Esterified Estrogens

Esterified estrogen is a plant-based product made from yams and soy. One study conducted by researchers at the University of California at San Francisco found that esterified estrogen didn't cause the increase in vaginal bleeding or buildup of the uterine walls—which is the precursor to endometrial cancer—that conjugated estrogens may. In fact, some researchers believe that you may not need to take a progestin or progesterone with this form of estrogen (since these are usually prescribed to fight against the possibility of endometrial cancer) or may be able to take a lower dose. Keep in mind, though, the prevailing evidence is there is an increased risk of endometrial cancer when taking unopposed estrogens.

Esterified estrogens are used to treat symptoms of menopause; deficiency in ovary function; some types of breast cancer in postmenopausal women; and vaginal atrophy.

Estratab is an esterfied estrogen tablet and is available in a 0.3, 0.625, and 2.5 mg daily dose. An important note: Estratab has been unavailable since spring 2001. Some sources say it will be reintroduced in the future, but it's unclear when this will happen. Keep in touch with your doctor or pharmacy, or contact the pharmaceutical company for more information.

Menest is an esterfied estrogen tablet in 0.3, 0.625, 1.25, and 2.5 mg doses and is administered in cycles, 3 weeks on and 1 week off. Monarch Pharmaceuticals, the manufacturer of Menest, states that "The lowest dose that will control symptoms should be chosen and medication should be discontinued as promptly as possible." Attempts to discontinue or taper medication should be made at 3- to 6-month intervals.

Do not take esterified estrogens without first talking to your doctor if you have a circulation, bleeding, or blood-clotting disorder; undiagnosed abnormal vaginal bleeding; or any type of breast, uterine, or hormone-dependent cancer.

Before taking esterified estrogens, tell your doctor if you have high blood pressure, angina, or heart disease; high levels of cholesterol or triglycerides in your blood; liver disease; kidney disease; asthma; epilepsy; migraines; diabetes; depression; gallbladder disease; uterine fibroids; or had a hysterectomy.

Possible side effects of esterified estrogens include an allergic reaction (difficulty breathing; closing of your throat; swelling of your lips, tongue, or face; or hives); a blood clot (pain, redness, and swelling in an arm or leg, shortness of breath, chest pain, headache, blurred vision, or confusion); a lump in a breast; or liver damage (yellowing of the skin or eyes, nausea, abdominal pain or discomfort, unusual bleeding or bruising, severe fatigue).

Other side effects may be more likely to occur: decreased appetite, nausea, or vomiting; swollen or tender breasts; acne or skin color changes;

decreased sex drive; migraine headaches or dizziness; water retention (swollen hands, feet, or ankles); problems with wearing contact lenses; depression; or changes in your menstrual cycle or breakthrough bleeding.

Before taking esterified estrogens, tell your doctor if you are taking any of the following medicines: an anticoagulant (blood thinner) such as warfarin (Coumadin); a thyroid medication such as Synthroid, Levoxyl, Levothroid, and others; insulin or an oral diabetes medicine such as glipizide (Glucotrol) or glyburide (DiaBeta, Micronase); tamoxifen (Nolvadex); didanosine (Videx); phenytoin (Dilantin) or ethotoin (Peganone); carbamazepine (Tegretol); phenobarbital (Solfoton, Luminal); primidone (Mysoline); or rifampin (Rifadin).

COMBINED THERAPY

When women began taking hormone replacement (HRT), they received estrogen only, known as estrogen replacement therapy, or ERT. As reports grew over increased rates of endometrial cancer among women on unopposed estrogen, doctors and pharmaceutical companies came up with the idea to add progestins for a few days in each cycle. This way, once the progestin was stopped, the uterus would shed its lining, thus eliminating the risk for cancer. This was the idea behind combined therapy.

However, two studies published in 2000 suggest that the addition of a progestin to estrogen in hormone therapy may actually *increase* the risk for breast cancer beyond that of estrogen alone. In light of these studies, doctors may need to reevaluate their risk-benefit analysis for prescribing combined HRT.

Estrogen and progesterone can be combined in various ways. In cyclical therapy, you take estrogen daily, add progestin for a few days of the month, and then stop the progestin. You'll get a period as soon as the progestin is stopped. Continuous therapy came about because many women complained about the bleeding. In this option, you take estrogen and progestin continuously, but use a lower dose of progestin. The thought is the continuous level of progestin will be too low to cause bleeding but high enough to block the stimulating effects of estrogen. While the continuous approach may cause less bleeding than the cyclical approach, it doesn't wholly eliminate the bleeding.

Combined Estradiol and Norgestinate

Ortho-Prefest is new form of HRT; it is made of estradiol, a bioidentical estrogen, and norgestimate, a synthetic progestin. Unlike other forms of continuous HRT which deliver both an estrogen and progestin every day, Ortho-Prefest has what's called a pulsatile delivery. In other words, there are two different pills—some with just estrogen and some with both estrogen and progestin. Every 3 days, you switch between the estrogen-only pills and estrogen plus progestin pills. So you're getting estrogen continuously, and progestin every 3 days for 3 days.

Many women find that they suffer more side effects from progestins, so by taking the progestin in this sequential manner, some women find the side effects minimized, and you're still getting enough progestin to balance out the estrogen and keep your uterine lining from building up too much.

Ortho-Prefest is used to treat the symptoms of menopause such as hot flashes; to treat vulvar and vaginal changes (itching, burning, dryness in or around the vagina, difficulty or burning with urination) caused by menopause. Standard dosage: 1 mg estradiol, 0.09 mg norgestimate (progestin delivered every 3 days for 3 days).

Do not take estradiol and norgestimate without first talking to your doctor if you have a circulation, bleeding, or blood-clotting disorder; undiagnosed abnormal vaginal bleeding; or any type of breast, uterine, or hormone-dependent cancer.

Before taking estradiol and norgestimate, tell your doctor if you have high blood pressure, angina, or heart disease; high levels of cholesterol or triglycerides in your blood; liver disease; kidney disease; asthma; epilepsy; migraines; depression; diabetes; gallbladder disease; uterine fibroids; or had a hysterectomy.

Possible side effects of estradiol and norgestimate include an allergic reaction (difficulty breathing, closing of your throat, swelling of your lips, tongue, or face, or hives); shortness of breath or pain in your chest; a painful, red, swollen leg; abnormal vaginal bleeding; pain, swelling, or tenderness in the abdomen; severe headache or vomiting; dizziness, faintness, or changes in vision or speech; yellowing of the skin or eyes; or a lump in a breast.

Other side effects may be more likely to occur, such as nausea and vomiting; tenderness or enlargement of the breasts; swelling of your hands or feet; spotty darkening of the skin, particularly on the face; changes in your menstrual cycle, such as irregular bleeding or spotting; headache, migraine, dizziness, faintness, or change in vision, including intolerance of contact lenses; depression; vaginal yeast infections; or enlargement of uterine fibroids.

Before taking estradiol and norgestimate, tell your doctor if you are taking any of the following medicines: insulin or an oral diabetes medicine such as glipizide (Glucotrol), glyburide (DiaBeta, Micronase, Glynase), chlorpropamide (Diabinese); tolazamide (Tolinase), tolbutamide (Orinase), and others; or an anticoagulant (blood thinner) such as warfarin (Coumadin).

Combined Estradiol and Norethindrone Acetate

Activella is one of the most recently introduced forms (approved in 2000) of HRT that combines both estrogen and progestin in one pill. Both the estrogen, which in this case is estradiol, and the progestin, which is norethrindrone acetate, are plant-based, but only the estrogen is bioidentical. (The combination of hormones is the same as in the CombiPatch, but of course Activella is in oral form, not patch form.) It's rather low-dose—on the low side of standard—which can be a good thing if you're wary of getting too much hormones. But on the flip side, it can also be a little too low for women who need higher amounts. The most commonly prescribed combination continuous HRT is Prempro, but the difference is with Activella you're getting estradiol, a plant-based estrogen, versus Premarin, an equine conjugated estrogen, in Prempro. Also the progestin in Activella is norethrindrone acetate—a synthetic plant form of progesterone that often causes fewer side effects than medroxyprogesterone acetate, which is in Prempro. Standard dosage: 1 mg estradiol and 0.5 mg norethindrone acetate daily for continuous therapy.

CombiPatch, introduced in late 1998, is notable because it is the first patch that delivers both estrogen and progesterone—more specifically, estradiol and norethindrone acetetate. Like the estrogen-only matrix patches, the CombiPatch is a thin, unobtrusive patch that delivers hormones through your skin. But because you get both estrogen and progestin from the patch, you don't have to take any pills in addition to using the patch; all you have to do is stick the patch on and change it twice a week. Standard dosage: .05 mg estradiol and .04 mg norethindrone acetate.

FemHRT is one of the newest forms of combination hormone replacement therapy offering both an estrogen and a progestin, but not the same ones as are in the commonly prescribed Prempro. The big difference between FemHRT and Prempro? The progestin in FemHRT is norethrindrone acetate, a synthetic form of progesterone that often causes fewer side effects than medroxyprogesterone acetate (MPA—most commonly sold under the brand name Provera). In addition, the estrogen in FemHRT isn't the conjugated estrogen Premarin, but ethinyl estradiol—the synthetic form of estrogen most commonly seen in birth control pills. Standard dosage: 5 mcg ethinyl estradiol, 1 mg norethindrone acetate.

Estradiol and norethindrone together are used to treat the symptoms of menopause such as hot flashes and to treat vulvar and vaginal changes (itching, burning, dryness in or around the vagina, difficulty or burning with urination) caused by menopause; and to replace estrogen in conditions such as hypogonadism, removal of the ovaries, or primary ovarian failure that result in a lack of estrogen.

Because it is a continuous form of HRT—that is, you take both estrogen and progestin daily—typically, after a few months, you stop having your period completely. In some women, this takes a little longer, and often, in the first few months, you may experience breakthrough bleeding.

Do not use estradiol and norethindrone without first talking to your doctor if you have a circulation, bleeding, or blood-clotting disorder; undiagnosed abnormal vaginal bleeding; any type of breast, uterine, or hormone-dependent cancer; or liver disease.

Before using estradiol and norethindrone, tell your doctor if you have high blood pressure, angina, or heart disease; high levels of cholesterol or triglycerides in your blood; kidney disease; asthma; epilepsy; migraines; depression; diabetes; gallbladder disease; uterine fibroids; or had a hysterectomy.

Possible side effects of estradiol and norethindrone are an allergic reaction (difficulty breathing, closing of your throat, swelling of your lips, tongue, or face, or hives); shortness or breath or pain in your chest; a painful, red, swollen leg; abnormal vaginal bleeding; pain, swelling, or tenderness in the abdomen; severe headache or vomiting, dizziness, faintness, or changes in vision or speech; yellowing of the skin or eyes; or a lump in a breast.

Other side effects may be more likely to occur, such as nausea and vomiting; tenderness or enlargement of the breasts; weakness; swelling of your hands or feet; spotty darkening of the skin, particularly on the face; difficulty in wearing contact lenses; vaginal irritation or discomfort; a rash or reaction at the patch application site; or changes in your menstrual cycle, painful menstruation, or breakthrough bleeding.

Before using estradiol and norethindrone, tell your doctor if you are taking an anticoagulant (blood thinner) such as warfarin (Coumadin). You may not be able to use estradiol and norethindrone, or you may require a dosage adjustment or special monitoring during your treatment if you are taking warfarin (Coumadin).

Esterified Estrogens and Methyltestosterone

This is a form of HRT that combines estrogen and testosterone in one pill. Remember, esterified estrogen is a plant-based product made from yams and soy. Methyltestosterone is a naturally occurring androgen that is produced in the testes in men and, in small amounts, by the ovaries and the brain in women. The most commonly prescribed brand is Estra-test, which contains esterified estrogens plus testosterone; however, Pre-marin is also available in a testosterone-included form.

Most research finds that testosterone is especially important for a woman who has undergone surgical menopause. When you have your ovaries removed, you aren't producing the tiny amount of testosterone that a woman with ovaries does even after menopause. So there is a good chance that you may suffer from more intense hot flashes and a loss of interest in sex. By replacing the testosterone in addition to estrogen, you may be able to lessen these symptoms.

A note of warning: Some studies have shown that testosterone may raise blood pressure. The important factor is the ratio of testosterone to estrogen, so if you do take Estratest or another testosterone in HRT, you should be sure to have your testosterone levels as well as your estrogen lev-els checked initially and tracked while you're on the HRT. Keep in mind testosterone still hasn't been studied closely, so it's difficult to be sure what the long-term side effects may be.

The major decision in this case is whether you'd prefer taking the natural estrogen in Estratest or the conjugated estrogen in Premarin with methyltestosterone. In addition, the Premarin plus testosterone has a much higher dosage of testosterone in it—over double the amount. Since many doctors advocate starting low with hormones, then building up if there's no effect, you may be better off opting for the Estratest. In addition, some doctors prescribe Estratest H.S. in conjunction with another estro-gen—you alternate between the two, so you get only half the dosage of the testosterone. In this way, you may be getting enough to help your prob-lems, but not more than your body needs . . . and not enough to run the risk of side effects.

Estratest, Estratest H.S., Menogen, and Menogen H.S. are all brand-name tablets that combine esterified estrogen and methyltestosterone.

This combination is used to treat vasomotor symptoms and diminished libido that have not responded to estrogen therapy alone. Standard dosage: Estratest / Menogen tablets contain 1.25 mg of esterified estrogens and 2.5 mg of methyltestosterone once or twice daily, cyclically for 3 weeks on and 1 week off. Estratest H.S./ Menogen H.S. are a half-strength option, containing 0.625 mg of esterified estrogens and 1.25 of methyltestosterone, once or twice day cyclically.

Do not take esterified estrogens and methyltestosterone without first talking to your doctor if you have a circulation, bleeding, or blood-clotting disorder; undiagnosed abnormal vaginal bleeding; or any type of breast, uterine, or hormone-dependent cancer.

Before taking esterified estrogens and methyltestosterone, tell your doctor if you have high blood pressure, angina, or heart disease; high levels of cholesterol or triglycerides in your blood; liver disease; kidney disease; asthma; epilepsy; migraines; diabetes; depression; gallbladder disease; uterine fibroids; or had a hysterectomy.

Possible side effects of esterified estrogens and methyltestosterone include an allergic reaction (difficulty breathing, closing of your throat, swelling of your lips, tongue, or face, or hives); a blood clot (pain, redness, and swelling in an arm or leg, shortness of breath, chest pain, headache, blurred vision, or confusion); a lump in a breast; liver damage (yellowing of the skin or eyes, nausea, abdominal pain or discomfort, unusual bleeding or bruising, severe fatigue); vomiting; or hoarseness, deepening of your voice, male pattern baldness, excessive hair growth, or clitoral enlargement (these changes may be irreversible).

Other side effects may be more likely to occur such as: decreased appetite or nausea; swollen breasts; acne or skin color changes; increased or decreased sex drive; migraine headaches or dizziness; water retention (swollen hands, feet, or ankles); intolerance to contact lenses; depression; or changes in your menstrual cycle or breakthrough bleeding.

Before taking esterified estrogens and methyltestosterone, tell your doctor if you are taking any of the following medicines: an anticoagulant (blood thinner) such as warfarin (Coumadin); a thyroid medication; insulin or another diabetes medicine such as glipizide (Glucotrol) or glyburide (DiaBeta, Micronase); tamoxifen (Nolvadex); a tricyclic antidepressant such as amitriptyline (Elavil), doxepin (Sinequan), nortriptyline (Pamelor), imipramine (Tofranil), and others; didanosine (Videx); phenytoin (Dilantin) or ethotoin (Peganone); carbamazepine (Tegretol); phenobarbital (Solfoton, Luminal); primidone (Mysoline); or rifampin (Rifadin).

Premarin with Methyltestosterone

Premarin and methyltestosterone combined are used to treat symptoms of menopause that have not responded to estrogen therapy alone. These are most often used to treat vasomotor symptoms of menopause and diminished libido. The standard dosage is 0.625 mg of Premarin and 5 mg of methyltestosterone once or twice daily for 3 weeks on and 1 week off. See the preceding sections for detailed information about Premarin and methyltestosterone.

Do not take Premarin and methyltestosterone without first talking to your doctor if you have a circulation, bleeding, or blood-clotting disorder; undiagnosed abnormal vaginal bleeding; or any type of breast, uterine, or hormone-dependent cancer.

Before taking Premarin and methyltestosterone, tell your doctor if you have high blood pressure, angina, or heart disease; high levels of cholesterol or triglycerides in your blood; liver disease; kidney disease; asthma; epilepsy; migraines; diabetes; depression; gallbladder disease; uterine fibroids; or had a hysterectomy.

Possible side effects of conjugated estrogens and methyltestosterone include an allergic reaction (difficulty breathing, closing of your throat, swelling of your lips, tongue, or face, or hives); a blood clot (pain, redness, and swelling in an arm or leg, shortness of breath, chest pain, headache, blurred vision, or confusion); a lump in a breast; liver damage (yellowing of the skin or eyes, nausea, abdominal pain or discomfort, unusual bleeding or bruising, severe fatigue); vomiting; or hoarseness, deepening of your voice, male pattern baldness, excessive hair growth, or clitoral enlargement (these changes may be irreversible).

Other effects may be more likely to occur, such as decreased appetite or nausea; swollen breasts; acne or skin color changes; increased or decreased sex drive; migraine headaches or dizziness; water retention (swollen hands, feet, or ankles); intolerance to contact lenses; depression; or changes in your menstrual cycle or breakthrough bleeding.

Before taking Premarin and methyltestosterone, tell your doctor if you are taking any of the following medicines: an anticoagulant (blood thinner) such as warfarin (Coumadin); a thyroid medication; insulin or another diabetes medicine such as glipizide (Glucotrol) or glyburide (DiaBeta, Micronase); tamoxifen (Nolvadex); a tricyclic antidepressant such as amitriptyline (Elavil), doxepin (Sinequan), nortriptyline (Pamelor), imipramine (Tofranil), and others; didanosine (Videx); phenytoin (Dilantin) or ethotoin (Peganone); carbamazepine (Tegretol); phenobarbital (Solfoton, Luminal); primidone (Mysoline); or rifampin (Rifadin).

Conjugated Estrogen and Medroxyprogesterone (MPA)

On July 9, 2002, the National Heart, Lung, and Blood Institute announced that it was stopping the Prempro study being performed as a part of the Women's Health Initiative. This study was conducted to assess whether long-term use of Prempro would reduce the risk of coronary heart disease in postmenopausal women. It was stopped early because the overall health risks of Prempro exceeded the benefits of the drug. The Women's Health Initiative (WHI) study found an increased risk of breast cancer, heart disease, nonfatal heart attacks, and blood clots in women taking conjugated estrogens and medroxyprogesterone long-term. In the light of this study, the makers of Prempro and Premphase, Wyeth, declared that women should be on these drugs for only the shortest amount of time possible.

These drugs were designed to make HRT as easy as possible—by combining both estrogen and a progestin in one tablet. Both Prempro and Premphase contain Premarin or Provera in the standard dosages you'd get if you took them individually. See the preceding sections for detailed information about Premarin and Provera.

Prempro and Premphase are used for treatment of moderate to severe vasomotor symptoms associated with the menopause and treatment of vulvar and vaginal atrophy. Standard dosage for Prempro is 0.625 conjugated estrogen/2.5 mg MPA, daily, for with Prempro, you take both estrogen and progestin every day—which emulates continuous therapy. With Premphase, estrogen is taken every day, and the progestin is added to the estrogen pill for the last two 2 weeks of the menstrual cycle. This is done so that it most closely resembles the normal menstrual cycle. Premphase contains .625 milligrams of Premarin and 2.5 milligrams of MPA; the progesterone is in only 2 weeks' worth of the pills.

Do not take conjugated estrogens and medroxyprogesterone without first talking to your doctor if you have a circulation, bleeding, or blood-clotting disorder; liver disease; undiagnosed abnormal vaginal bleeding; or any type of breast, uterine, or hormone-dependent cancer.

Before taking conjugated estrogens and medroxyprogesterone, tell your doctor if you have high blood pressure, angina, or heart disease; high levels of cholesterol or triglycerides in your blood; kidney disease; asthma; epilepsy; migraines; depression; diabetes; gallbladder disease; uterine fibroids; or had a hysterectomy.

Possible side effects of conjugated estrogens and medroxyprogesterone include an allergic reaction (difficulty breathing, closing of your throat, swelling of your lips, tongue, or face, or hives); a blood clot (pain, redness, and swelling in an arm or leg, shortness of breath, coughing blood, chest pain, headache, blurred vision; or confusion); unusual or abnormal vaginal bleeding; pain, swelling, or tenderness in the abdomen; liver damage (yellowing of the skin or eyes, nausea, abdominal pain or discomfort, unusual bleeding or bruising, severe fatigue); or a lump in a breast.

Other, less serious side effects may be more likely to occur: changes in appetite or weight, swelling of your hands or feet, tiredness or weakness, irregular bleeding or spotting, depression, an increase in body or facial hair or hair loss, swollen or tender breasts, nausea, headache or insomnia, changes in your voice, or areas of darker skin.

Before taking conjugated estrogens and medroxyprogesterone, tell your doctor if you are taking any of the following medicines: insulin or an oral diabetes medicine such as glipizide (Glucotrol), glyburide (DiaBeta, Micronase, Glynase), chlorpropamide (Diabinese), tolazamide (Tolinase), tolbutamide (Orinase), and others; aminoglutethimide (Cytadren);

an anticoagulant (blood thinner) such as warfarin (Coumadin); calcium supplements; or estradiol and medroxyprogesterone.

DIETARY SUPPLEMENTS

Just as Dorothy, Toto, the Scarecrow, the Tin Man, and the Lion leave the forest and the Emerald City of Oz is in their sight, they pass through a beautiful poppy field. Something mysterious begins to happen and they start to get tired. The Wicked Witch is watching from her crystal ball as the poppies put them all to sleep, thereby delaying their arrival in Oz and giving the witch more time to get those slippers. Who would have thought this beautiful field of flowers could be so powerful? It reminds us not to forget the power of natural elements such as flowers and plants, which are found in dietary supplements, another option many women take.

Within one week of the Women's Health Initiative announcement, sales were up for black cohosh, a botanical remedy used by Algonquian natives for centuries to ease the symptoms of menopause. GlaxoSmith-Kline, makers of Remifemin, a black cohosh preparation, normally pitched the botanical only to 9,000 obstetrician-gynecologists; that week they began passing out information to 28,000 internists and family practitioners. Six weeks of free drug samples were snapped up in two.

Menopausal women already spend about $600 million annually on alternative treatments for menopause, according to the National Center for Complementary and Alternative Medicine. But the possible turn to alternative medicine therapies for menopause may raise as many questions as it answers. Numerous dietary supplements—the legal name for herbal, botanical, vitamin, and mineral products used to prevent or treat symptoms—are sold for relief of the hot flashes and mood changes that often accompany menopause. Supplements are neither food nor drugs, so manufacturers do not have to provide any evidence to support purported benefits before marketing their products. This means supplements are not held to the same standard of testing the FDA requires of prescription drugs. Nor do all manufacturers meet standards of good manufacturing procedures. Products coming out of production facilities may vary greatly in the amount of the purported plant constituents, or active ingredients, in the few cases we do know the active ingredients. Recently the botanical industry set up voluntary guidelines, and some manufacturers have signed agreements in kind affirming that they will produce products set to an industry-defined standard. However, without mandatory oversight, problems of adulteration, contamination, and dose standardization will continue. In the list of products below, general dosage recommendations are given but are not meant as a guide for how you should use these products. It is just to give you a general idea of the frequency and amounts some products call for. While herbal products on the market may look similar or have similar-sounding names, their ingredients could be very different, so do not assume that dosage instructions for one can be interchanged for another.

The best studied and most popular for menopausal problems are black cohosh, soy extracts, and red clover. The latter two contain phytoestrogens, chemical compounds that function in some ways like estrogen, the main hormone of femaleness. The National Center for Complementary and Alternative Medicine at the National Institutes of Health is funding two clinical trials for black cohosh. One is a head-to-head study of HRT, black cohosh, red clover, and a placebo at the University of Illinois at Chicago. Over the next year, 112 women will take part in the randomized trial and be followed for a year. That trial may help answer questions about the botanicals' effectiveness, but it is not likely to answer questions about long-term safety. The second clinical trial is being conducted at Columbia University College of Physicians and Surgeons. This year-long randomized controlled trial of black cohosh versus placebo is designed to look at long-term safety.

For women choosing a more natural or botanical choice to menopausal changes, plant-derived hormones (phytoestrogens and phytosterols) have become increasingly popular in this country. Plants do not make estrogens in the classic sense of the term. Plants make sterol molecules; these compounds, phytoestrogens, when consumed, are converted by our bodies into substances that act like estrogens. These plant compounds also form the basis of the natural hormones that are synthesized in the lab. Natural hormones cannot be changed in the body from their wild form to the identical estrogen or progesterone forms.

Keep in mind that not all herbs are equal. They can counteract each other and should not be taken in conjunction with prescription hormones. Everyone can have an individual reaction to supplements, just as with foods and drugs; try one at a time or wait before adding a second. If you have had cancer, beware of using herbs with phytoestrogens. It is not yet known if supplements with phytoestrogens are powerful enough to cause a recurrence.

Black cohosh is made from the root nodules of a North American plant in the buttercup family. Also sold under the name Remifemin, it is used to relieve hot flashes and vaginal dryness. Black cohosh extract is one of the leading botanicals sold in Germany and is the country's top-selling menopausal herbal remedy. However, the German Commission E, a governmental regulatory group, recommends the use of any black cohosh product for not more than six months, since data on long-term safety are not yet available. Possible, though rare, side effects are nausea or vomiting and uterine contractions. Some studies, however, indicate that like estrogen, black cohosh may increase cell proliferation. Most recommendations are that you take black cohosh extract that contains either 20 or 40 mg twice a day. We do not know how black cohosh works to decrease hot flashes.

Don quai, dang gui, and tang kuei are different names of the same plant. They are all types of angelicas. They are used to relieve hot flashes and claim to improve circulation. It is the most prescribed Chinese herbal medicine for menopausal problems. Angelicas supposedly regulate and balance the menstrual cycle and are said to strengthen the uterus. Possible side effects are anticoagulation and photosensitivity. Most of the benefit of angelica is thought to result from the fact that it's a coumarin, which is a type of compound that decreases blood clotting. The recommended dosage is 10 to 40 drops of the fresh root daily. You should not take angelicas if you have heavy menstrual bleeding, take blood-thinning drugs, or have fibroids.

Ginseng is a plant whose root is used medicinally. There are different species that grow in different countries. It is used to balance stress, improve circulation, and stimulate the immune system. Ginseng is reputed to be an aphrodisiac, a claim unsubstantiated by medical evidence. Side effects are hypertension, anxiety, depression, and insomnia.

Vitex, also known as agnus-castus or chasteberry, comes from the chaste tree in the Mediterranean. It affects the pituitary gland and stimulates the release of the three hormones: luteinizing hormone (LH), follicle-stimulating hormone (FSH), and prolactin. It seems to normalize progesterone levels. Vitex is generally used for loss of libido and vaginal dryness. Claims are that using vitex regularly for a few months will increase your natural levels of progesterone and help control hot flashes, depression, and vaginal atrophy. Most recommendations call for 1 capsule up to 3 times daily or 10 to 30 drops of extract in juice or water up to 3 times daily.

Valerian is a root extract and is used as a calming agent, for mood disturbances, and to relieve insomnia. The active ingredient has never been identified but is thought to be gamma amino butyric acid (GABA) derivative. Similar GABA-like compounds have been found in chamomile, which is also used as an herbal sleep aid. Valerian is recommended to be taken in capsule form, 2 grams 2 hours before bedtime and 2 grams at bedtime. Some labels warn not to take it continuously for more than 2 weeks.

Licorice is a perennial herb. It is one of the most extensively used and scientifically investigated herbal medicines. Licorice is said to regulate the ratio of estrogen to progesterone. It is usually taken for vaginal dryness and mood swings in doses of $1/4$ teaspoon of extract twice a day. Some women have reported success using it to treat hot flashes. A cautionary note: In large doses licorice has been reported to raise blood pressure and cause electrolyte disturbances.

Soy contains phytoestrogens, plant-based isoflavones that are the slightly weaker cousins of estrogen. Soy is purported to take the edge off hot flashes, but doctors say its effect is nowhere near estrogen's. The effects of soy protein found in whole foods, soy protein isolates, and those of isoflavone isolates made into powders or pills may not be all the same. Even soy foods are not necessarily reliable sources of biologically active isoflavones. Although the mechanisms of action of soy and dietary isoflavones are not fully understood, they appear to involve binding to the estrogen receptor. For this reason, one should not assume these dietary supplements are safe for women with estrogen-dependent cancers—most important, breast cancer. You can get soy from a variety of sources—including soy milk, tofu, roasted soy nuts, tempeh, soybeans, even products that are made to taste like other foods (like soy hot dogs, soy cheese, and soy ice cream). High amounts of soy isoflavones can affect your thyroid, so if you have thyroid disease, speak with your doctor before using soy as a symptom reliever.

St. John's wort is made from extracts of the flower *Hypericum perforatum* and has been used for centuries to treat mild to moderate depression. Recent research has indicated that the herb's antidepressive effect may be largely due to its ability to inhibit the reuptake of serotonin, a process mimicked by such synthetic antidepressants as Prozac and Zoloft. The generally recommended dose is 1 capsule 3 times a day. Side effects can include dry mouth, dizziness, and constipation. This is not to be used with other antidepressants.

Red clover is another plant that contains phytoestrogens and is also high in bioflavonoids. Like the other phytoestrogen-containing plants, red clover has been reported to reduce hot flashes and generally minimize other menopausal symptoms. There are many red clover products on the market.

Evening primrose produces seeds rich in gamma-linolenic acid (GLA) and contains several anticoagulant substances. It is commonly recommended for premenstrual syndrome, menopausal symptoms, and bladder symptoms.

Garden sage is a relative of the sage plant containing bioflavonoids and phytosterols, so it's a weak estrogen and has some progestogenic effects. It is used to treat excessive sweating, night sweats, mood swings, and headaches. The recommended dosage is 1 to 2 spoonfuls of dried leaf infusion 1 to 8 times daily as a tea.

THAT'S A HORSE OF A DIFFERENT COLOR

Dorothy, Toto, the Scarecrow, the Tin Man, and the Lion all awaken in the poppy field with the Emerald City in their sight. They arrive to find a large door and no way inside the city, so they knock. A small man peers through a opening in the door and asks what they want. Dorothy says they're here to see the wizard, but the man says no one sees the wizard. Neither the distance they've traveled nor their pleading sways the gate-keeper's mind until the Scarecrow points out that Dorothy is wearing the ruby slippers. A smile breaks across the gatekeeper's face and he exclaims, "The ruby slippers. Well, why didn't you say so? That's a horse of a different color." Those mysterious and magical ruby slippers opened another door for Dorothy. Just like Dorothy keeps trying different tactics each time the gatekeeper slams the door in her face, women need to remember to try different options as well. Some women who have asked for hormone or dietary supplements and haven't felt relief are looking into the use of drugs traditionally used to treat depression for their menopausal symptoms.

During the past decade, treatment of depression has been revolutionized by selective serotonin reuptake inhibitors, or SSRIs, a class of compounds now one of the most prescribed in the world. Prozac, Paxil, Luvox, Zoloft, and Celexa are examples of available SSRIs.

SSRIs work by allowing the body to make the best use of the reduced amounts of serotonin that it has at the time. The brain is made up of millions of interconnected brain cells (neurons). Messages travel along these cells like electricity down a wire, but when the message reaches the end of the neuron, it has to jump a gap (synapse) to the next cell or group of cells. This is achieved by the neuron releasing tiny amounts of a chemical (neurotransmitter) into the gap between the nerve cells. The receiving neuron has many places on its surface that act like locks, for which the appropriate neurotransmitter is the key. These are called receptors. When enough of the neurotransmitter has locked onto these receptors, a nerve impulse is started in the new nerve, and thus the message gets from one nerve to the next.

In order to allow the nerve to recover and receive the next message, and in order to replenish stocks of the neurotransmitter in the original neuron, so it can be ready to send the next message, the body has a clever way of removing the neurotransmitter from the receptors and allowing it to be taken back into the originating nerve; this is called reuptake.

In depression, certain neurotransmitters are relatively lacking; one of those is serotonin. The SSRIs (selective serotonin reuptake inhibitors) slow down the process of returning the serotonin to the end of the neuron it comes from. This leads to the chemical remaining in the vicinity of the receptors for longer, making it more likely that enough will build up to set off the impulse in the next neuron. In due course, the levels of natural serotonin will rise again, and the SSRI can be reduced and withdrawn.

So if SSRIs were developed to treat depression, you might wonder how and why they are now used to treat symptoms of menopause. SSRIs were initially studied for hot flashes because of anecdotal reports by women who were placed on SSRIs for depression and noticed a lessening of premenstrual symptoms and hot flashes. So what's the link between SSRIs and hot flashes? Well, the recent thinking is that estrogen withdrawal might be associated with a decline in circulating serotonin. This decline in serotonin increases the sensitivity of the hypothalamic receptor regulating your body temperature. So an external trigger, such as a change in ambient temperature, or an internal trigger, such as immediate changes in hormones, can result in imbalances of various neurotransmitters and stimulation of the hypothalamic receptor that controls body temperature, resulting in the sensation of the hot flash. If you have had a hot flash you know while the threshold between sweating and shivering is wide in pre-menopausal women, it is quite narrow in menopausal women and is easily triggered.

Recent randomized clinical trials have supported the use of SSRIs to manage hot flashes. Venlafaxine reduced hot flashes by 60 percent compared with a 20 percent reduction in patients who received placebo, and fluoxetine did so by 50 percent compared with 36 percent on placebo. Preliminary results suggested that sertraline was no more effective than placebo in decrease in hot flashes. In a study of 165 menopausal women, a six-week treatment with paroxetine controlled-release 12.5 mg or 25.0 mg daily was associated with a median reduction of 62 percent and 65 percent in hot flash score, respectively, compared with a 38 percent reduction for placebo.

Some recent trials comparing SSRIs, St. John's wort, and placebo have shown surprisingly little difference among the three. In these trials, sponsored by manufacturers, placebo and St. John's wort were close in effectiveness, while the prescription drugs fared very slightly better.

This phenonemon of the placebo effect is not new and has been found in the area of estrogen treatment as well. A most provocative placebo trial on estrogen was reported by Dr. Jean Coope in the *British Medical Journal* in 1975. All of the volunteers had menopausal symptoms. Half received conjugated estrogens while the others got lactose (milk sugar) pills. All were monitored for the following complaints: insomia, nervousness, depression, dizziness, weakness, joint pain, headaches, palpitations, prickling sensations, and hot flashes. The first ninety days of the study brought dramatic improvement for both groups. There was no significant difference in any symptom, except that the placebo did not relieve the hot flashes as completely.

Then midway through the six-month study, the products were switched, with interesting results. The real estrogen pills maintained the favorable response first brought about by the dummy medication, but the group that had first been treated with estrogen experienced a pronounced return of symptoms when the placebo was substituted. Thus, taking the first estrogen pill may be a major decision. Contrary to assurances that it can be used for a few months and then terminated, many women may have to endure cold turkey if they drop it abruptly. Coope's study has raised questions rarely addressed in public on whether estrogens are addictive to some users.

If you decide to look into SSRI treatment, please make sure your doctor knows of any other medication you are taking. SSRIs may not be compatible with all hormone or herbal supplements. And even in light of recent studies, several questions remain unanswered. Which, if any, of the many SSRIs is preferable? Are lower doses as effective against hot flashes as the doses recommended for depression? How long should patients take SSRIs, since hot flashes are generally short-lived?

I'M MELTING!

Once Dorothy and her friends get in to see the great and all-powerful Wizard of Oz, he makes demands of them before he will grant their requests. Dorothy must bring him the broomstick of the wicked Witch of the West. This seems impossible. Meek, kind Dorothy must kill the wicked witch to get her broom. So the four set out to where the witch lives when suddenly Dorothy is picked up by flying monkeys and whisked away to the witch's castle. Dorothy, alone and scared, does not know what to do while the witch tries to find a way to get those ruby slippers off Dorothy's feet. Thankfully, a sympathetic guard tells Dorothy the witch can be killed by pouring a bucket of water over her. So sweet and gentle Dorothy summons up all of her strength, and the next time the witch comes for her she throws the bucket of water over the witch. The witch screams and smoke pours out of her as she starts melting into the ground. Remembering that in our story the witch is the pharmaceutical companies, you can almost hear them screaming "Our profits are shrinking!" from the water that was doused on them when the WHI study was halted in the summer of 2002.

So where did meek little Dorothy from Kansas get the strength to kill the wicked witch? Some might say it's the testosterone, the so-called male hormone, giving Dorothy her nerve and aggression. There is growing evidence that decreased levels of testosterone may contribute to bone loss, fatigue, and vaginal dryness, so pharmaceutical companies are developing testosterone products for women. Remember, we earlier discussed combined estrogen and testosterone treatment, but this is important to include because while there are no testosterone-only products that are FDA approved for women now, these will most likely be available in the next few years.

That does not, however, mean that women cannot receive testosterone-only treatment now. Women are reporting that their gynecologists are prescribing testosterone treatments for them that are currently available for men. Let's be very clear about this: the products available on the market now are not—repeat, not—approved to be used by women by the FDA. This usually means that dosages have been set for men's bodies; side effects that may happen to women are not known and long-term effects have yet to be documented. Also bear in mind that it took years of research to produce information on the effects of estrogen supplements in women, so it will be quite some time before the literature on testosterone treatment catches up. What follows is a brief review of the available products as well as a look ahead to some projects in the pipeline.

In general, testosterone treatment is being looked into for women who have sexual dysfunction, have had their ovaries removed, or have Addison's disease or a disorder of the pituitary gland or hypothalamus. This is because testosterone is produced by the ovaries and adrenal gland; so if your ovaries were removed or you have Addison's disease, in which the adrenal glands don't function, or a glandular disorder that affects the ovaries or adrenals, you may not naturally produce the levels of testosterone your body needs.

AndroGel and Testim are testosterone gels and Androderm and Testoderm are testosterone patches approved only for use by men because the testosterone dose is too high for women. These products are used to fight conditions associated with low testosterone in men—fatigue, depression, low libido, reduced strength, and erectile dysfunction.

Watson Laboratories, Inc., the manufacturer of Androderm, describe their product in this way: "Testosterone gels and patches deliver physiologic amounts of testosterone producing circulating testosterone concentrations that approximate the normal rhythm of healthy young men. Androderm (testosterone transdermal system) delivers testosterone, the primary androgenic hormone. Testosterone is responsible for the normal growth and development of the male sex organs and for maintenance of secondary sex characteristics. These effects include the growth and maturation of the prostate, seminal vesicles, penis, and scrotum; development of male hair distribution, such as facial, pubic, chest, and axillary hair; laryngeal enlargement; vocal cord thickening; and alterations in body musculature and fat distribution." So this product gives you the testosterone level of a "healthy young man," and helps to deepen your voice and grow facial and chest hair. When considering taking a drug which is approved for use only by men, keep these considerations in mind.

Here is some important information straight from the manufacturers of these products: Testosterone topical is not approved for use by women and must not be used by women. Testosterone topical is in the FDA pregnancy category X. This means that testosterone topical will cause birth defects in an unborn baby. Pregnant women should avoid skin contact with the testosterone topical gel application site in men. Topical testosterones are so potent that women exposed to the gel their partner applies can develop male-pattern baldness, excessive body hair growth, a significant increase in acne, or menstrual irregularities. Do not use testosterone topical if you have cancer of the breast or prostate. Testosterone can worsen cancers of these types.

But since women are experimenting with the use of male-approved testosterone, some pharmaceutical companies have caught on and are now in the process of developing their own testosterone products for women. The only testosterone drug for menopausal symptoms on the horizon is LibiGel. LibiGel is being developed as a once-daily gel for treatment of menopausal women to treat hot flashes, vaginal atrophy, and lowered sex drive. This drug is still in its testing phase and needs the FDA's final stamp of approval before it can go to market. But remember, even if more testosterone products are made available for women, it can take years to really understand what these hormones do to our bodies—as we're learning with estrogen treatment. So sometimes it's better to wait and see how a new product fares than to be the first in line.

THE WIZARD'S NOT A WIZARD AFTER ALL

Finally Dorothy, Toto, the Scarecrow, Tin Man, and the Lion are in the presence of the great and all-powerful Wizard of Oz. As they cower before the giant floating head with a booming voice, Toto runs off and starts tugging on the curtain. He pulls it back to reveal a man shouting into a microphone. The giant head tells them to ignore the man behind the curtain, but Dorothy realizes the wizard is not really a wizard after all. The little man behind the curtain explains that he created the great wizard to have power in Oz. There is no wizard who can magically transport Dorothy home. Many women today are beginning to see that their doctors are not wizards; in many instances they are hiding behind a curtain of power which they and the drug industry have for years worked behind to maintain power over women. With the WHI announcement and others calling for the reevaluation of hormone replacement therapy, the curtain surrounding menopause is being drawn back. Perhaps women will be able to demedicalize menopause—take it back as a natural part of life, not a disease to be rid of.

But Dorothy is still in Oz and has no idea how to get home until Glinda appears to tell Dorothy she had the power to go home all along: the ruby slippers. Glinda tells Dorothy she had the power within herself the whole time, and Dorothy begins to realize it's true. No wonder the witch, our pharmaceutical companies, wanted the slippers so badly. The slippers were the key Dorothy needed to unlock the information she had all along. Dorothy realized ultimately that she had the power to help herself, just as all women do. By taking the initiative to become informed, you take the control away from the drug companies. Their biggest fear is that we will become educated consumers and stop accepting their products and claims about them as gospel. Talk to your friends and read books put out by authors and organizations not paid for by the drug industry. The internet has a multitude of websites devoted to women discussing their menopausal treatments. And most of all, listen to yourself; don't let anyone talk you into something you're not comfortable doing.

NOTES

Note 1.
Page 1, Paragraph 2
Surprise expressed by doctor friend . . .

Doctors need not have been taken so much off guard, as bad news on estrogens had been published in a rapid-fire series of important studies, beginning on January 25, 2000, when the National Cancer Institute revealed that the progestins needed to prevent cancer "down there" (in the uterus) increased the risk of cancer "up top" (in the breast.) *The Journal of the American Medical Association (JAMA)* carried an editorial called "Postmenopausal Estrogens—Opposed, Unopposed or None of the Above." It concluded, "It is time to reassess the commonly held belief that aging routinely requires pharmacological management." This was two and a half years before the bombshell of July 9, 2002.

One and a half years before the bombshell, in December 2000, when Dr. Tim Johnson announced the top medical breakthroughs of 2000 on *Good Morning America*, he included "the negative finding that long-term hormones do not work as claimed . . . Some treatments," he continued, "turn out to be less effective than they were considered originally. A number of studies this year showed that these drugs increased risk for breast cancer and weren't as effective in preventing heart disease as doctors had hoped."

Three months before the bombshell, on March 22, 2002, at an NIH meeting hosted by Dr. Vivian Pinn of the Office of Research on Women's Health, scientists from the Women's Health Initiative (WHI), met to give doctors and some reporters a preview of a book they'd been working on for seven years. It was called *International Position Paper on Women's Health and Menopause: A Comprehensive Approach* (NIH Publication No. 02-3284). Overall, this 298-page report is cautious on the benefits of estrogen compared to the risks, and also explains how new discoveries of hitherto unknown estrogen receptors in the female body have cast doubt on old theories of how estrogen products work.

During the two-and-a-half-year interval when scientific faith in estrogen declined, public confusion came from the fact that the downside studies alternated with positive news, much of the latter from sources that were less objective. Worried patients were often counseled by their doctors to carry on as before. "These reports tell you one thing this week, and the opposite next week." True enough, but in the opinion of the AMA, such advice tended to come from doctors who were too busy to separate the science from the fluff. So the AMA decided to "change all that." It put out two manuals and a CD known as the *User's Guide to the Medical Literature*. As coeditor Drummond Rennie, M.D., wrote in the Foreword, "It's designed to . . . free the clinician from practicing by rote, by guesswork . . . to put a stop to clinicians being ambushed by drug company representatives, or by their patients telling them of new therapies the clinicians are unable to evaluate. To end their dependence on out-of-date authority. To enable the practitioner to work with the patient and use the literature as a tool to solve the patient's problems. . . ." (Gordon Guyatt, M.D., and Drummond Rennie, M.D., Eds., *User's Guide to the Medical Literature: A Manual for Evidence Based Clinical Practice*. Chicago: AMA Press, 2002)

Note 2.
Page 5, Paragraph 4

On the one hand many prestigious doctors have noted the escalating influence that the pharmaceutical industry appears to hold over medical research and practice. For example, in the issue of *JAMA* for January 21, 2003, a group from the Yale University School of Medicine reported that "About one fourth of biomedical investigations at academic institutions have some affiliation with industry, whose support of biomedical research increased dramatically in the last two decades. . . . Industry's share of total investment in biomedical research and development grew from approximately 32 percent in 1980 to 62% in 2000. . . . This review shows that financial relationships are pervasive and problematic." In a *Washington Post* Op-Ed published June 20, 2001, Drs. Marcia Angell and Arnold Relman, former editors-in-chief of the *New England Journal of Medicine (NEJM)*, lamented that: "Last year drug companies spent more than $8 billion and employed 83,000 sales representatives to woo doctors. They provided them with gifts, meals and trips, as well as another $8 billion worth of free drug samples. The companies fund and thereby influence much of the continuing medical education doctors need to renew their licenses, and they handsomely support the scientific meetings of medical societies, where they hawk their wares and also sponsor their own programs."

On the other hand there are equally prestigious doctors taking the side of industry, who, following the halting of the Prempro trial, made themselves available to encourage doctors and patients to switch to other products or other delivery systems, particularly the transdermal patch. Many women say they are changing over to the patch because they have heard that in this form estrogen is "easier on the liver," and thus "safer." But it may not be true. Like so many claims for estrogen, there's a plausible theory but no persuasive research. The FDA, the American College of Obstetrics and Gynecology (ACOG), the North American Menopause Society (NAMS), and even Wyeth itself have agreed that boxed warning labels, like those on Prempro, must be placed *on all products containing estrogen*, and must advise that the drugs may slightly increase the risk of heart attacks, strokes, blood clots, and breast cancer. Specifically the FDA said, "It must be assumed that all other products containing estrogen, including patches, creams and pills, have similar problems unless proved otherwise."

Small clinical trials comparing the patch with placebo indicate, so far, that, as with similar oral products, heart attacks are increased *not* decreased. One such study of 255 women by S. C. Clark and his associates appeared in the *British Journal of Obstetrics and Gynecology* 2002; 109: 1056–1062: Conclusion: "Despite the small sample size, there was a troubling 30% increase in risk for acute coronary syndromes in the active treatment arm."

Thus, on January 9, 2003, Dr. Isaac Schiff, the gynecologist who headed the ACOG task force that urged members not to assume that other estrogen formulations were safer than Prempro, complained to Gina Kolata of the *New York Times* that "some distinguished people in my discipline, I am embarrassed to say, put out a letter saying the patch is safer."

They certainly did. I have a copy of the letter. I applaud Dr. Schiff for his courage in calling their bluff. They are six eminent professors, departmental chairs, deans, influential authors, and editors, who call themselves the Women's Health Advisory Board on the letterhead. Their letter to gynecologists is dated September 18, 2002. Their recommendation is to "stop Premarin for long term use" and to "initiate or replace oral hormonal therapy with transdermal 17B estradiol in the lowest effective dose for each individual woman." They do not say who has funded them, nor do they present proof that the patch is safer, but they state that "it is imperative that we counter this panic reaction" (to the "confusion and media turmoil stimulated by the WHI announcement on July 9th"). The message of this letter, as I read it, is: "You can tell your patients; 'and now for something completely different—the patch'—and thereby get them to stay on hormones." The letter is signed by Dr. Nathan Kase "for the HAB."

Dr. Kase is Professor at the Department of Obstetrics and Gynecology at Mt. Sinai School of Medicine in New York, former Dean at Mt. Sinai, and former Chair of Obstetrics and Gynecology at Yale. Following him on the masthead is Dr. Daniel R. Mishell, Professor, and Chairman of the Department of Obstetrics and Gynecology at the School of Medicine at the University of Southern California. The third is Dr. Leon Speroff, Professor of Obstetrics and Gynecology at the Oregon Health and Science University School of Medicine, and an influential author. Next is Dr. Sarah Berga, a researcher of considerable standing at the University of Pittsburgh, and in fifth place, Dr. Mary Lake Polan, Professor and Chairman of the Department of Gynecology and Obstetrics at the Stanford University School of Medicine. The highly educated Dr. Polan possesses an M.D, a Ph.D., and an M.PH., and she was one of eleven doctors, scientists, and other experts named by HHS Secretary Tommy Thompson to the Secretary's Advisory Committee on Human Research Protection. She has also served on the board of Wyeth, accepted major funding from Ethicon, a division of Johnson & Johnson, to finance an endoscopic laboratory run by Dr. Carman Nezhat, the famous but controversial fertility doctor. She has also been criticized for praising such questionable products as AginMax, an herbal aphrodisiac for women, produced by Mountain View's Daily Wellness Company where Dr. Polan has served as medical director, according to a July 5, 2001, report in the *San Jose Metro*. The sixth listed member of the Women's Health Advisory Board is Dr. Irwin Rosenberg at Tufts. The email address on the transdermal campaign letter (info@whab.org) is inoperative, but a press release issued by Women First Healthcare, a specialty pharmaceutical company based in San Diego, states that Dr. Nathan Kase is Chairman of the Women First Health Advisory Board, and that on their behalf he held a conference call on July 11, 2002, to discuss the Women's Health Initiative findings. According to their website (www.womenfirst. com), "The mission of Women First is to help midlife women make informed choices regarding their health care and to provide pharmaceutical products—the Company's primary liberating experience. Others think of it as a negative event. In the developed world the percentage of women over 50 years of age has tripled in the last 100 years. Due to a reduction in mortality and a decrease in birthrate the female life expectancy, which was 50 years in 1900, is 81.7 today.

From: *Women's Health and Menopause: A Comprehensive Approach.* (NIH publication No. 02-3284 July 2002.)

Note 8.
Page 9, Paragraph 2

George H. Napheys, *The Physical Life of Woman: Advice to the Maiden, Wife, and Mother.* (Canada, 1881).

An interesting website for further reading on the history of menopause can be found in Canada, at http://www.geocities.com/menobeyond/

Note 9.
Page 10, Paragraph 1

The Diseases of Females by Thomas Graham, cited by Madeline Gray in *The Changing Years.* (New York: Doubleday, 1951.)

Note 10.
Page 11, Paragraph 2

Brown-Sequard's lecture translated by Madeline Gray, *The Changing Years* (op.cit.)

Note 11.
Page 12, Paragraph 3

A Brown University anatomy student named Edgar Allen

Edgar Allen (b. May 2, 1892, Canyon City, Colorado. d. Feb. 3, 1943, New Haven, Conn.) was a leading authority on the mechanisms of sex hormones, discovered oestrogen and investigated the hormonal mechanisms that control the female reproductive cycle. Along with Edward Doisy he developed the Allen-Doisy test to determine oestrogen content. He served as professor of anatomy and Dean of the medical school at the University of Missouri before returning to the east coast as professor of anatomy and Chairman of the Department of the Yale School of Medicine 1933–43.

From: www.whonamedit.com/doctor

Note 12.
Page 14, Paragraph 2

Allen was getting more into research on the role of estrogens in female cancers.

Allen was among the early scientific geniuses who understood—eighty years before the mouse and human genomes were completed and compared—that, in the words of genome scientist Allan Bradley from the Sanger Institute in England (*Nature* Magazine, December 5, 2002), "The mouse has so many parallels with humans. Detailed analysis of organs, tissues, and cells reveal many similarities, including whole organ systems, reproduction, behavior, and disease. The mouse is an excellent surrogate for exploring human biology." It is now official that 99% of mouse genes match human. It was Allen whose hunch that in female reproduction the species were identical which laid the groundwork for the Greatest Experiment.

But think about the history, the most creative, the four most imposing figures, the A, B, C and D of estrogen research. Allen, (Edgar) Butenandt, (Adolph) Collip, (James) and Dodds (E. Charles) all fretted about the cancers that the estrogens they developed were bringing out in mice. Their friends and followers in the cancer-research communities pursued their own experiments and tended to concur. But those who wished to profit from the estrogen products dismissed the relevance of the "mouse work" and won the day. Had it been possible, in the 1930s, to map and compare the mouse and human genomes, estrogen products would have been reserved for special situations, not marketed off-handedly, and the Greatest Experiment would not have taken place.

Note 13.
Page 15, Paragraph 5
had been reported by Dr. Saul Gusberg in 1947
    S.B. Gusberg, "Precursors of corpus carcinoma: estrogens and adenomatous hyperplasia" *American Journal of Obstetrics and Gynecology.* 54:905–926 (1947).

CHAPTER 2: FOUNTAIN OF YOUTH OR GOLDEN FLEECE?

COLLIP SECTION

Note 14.
Page 17, Paragraph 1
    Madeline Gray, *The Changing Years.* New York: Doubleday. 1951, 1957, 1967, 1980, etc.

Note 15.
Page 18, Paragraph 2
Biochemist James Bertram "Bert" Collip
    James Bertram Collip (b. November 20, 1892 in Bellville, Ontario. d. June 19, 1965 in London, Ontario) was one of the great minds of Canadian medicine. Graduating from Trinity College, Toronto, at age 15, completed doctorate in biochemistry. At University of Alberta had outstanding career in biochemical research. He was on a traveling fellowship when he accepted the invitation of the University of Toronto to work with Banting and Best on the development of insulin. His efforts at purifying insulin by using the bovine pancreas, produced insulin in a form that permitted clinical use. Completing an MD, Dr. Collip accepted the chair of Biochemistry at McGill, where he launched into an extensive study of hormones. In 1941 he became Chairman of McGill's new Institute of Endocrinology. Dr. Collip capped a brilliant career as Dean of Medicine at the University of Western Ontario.
    From: Canadian Medical Hall of Fame at www.cdnmedhall.org

Note 16.
Page 18, Paragraph 3
As of this writing, some eighty years have passed, but Canadians still talk about
    "In life, James Bertram Collip was never properly recognized for his role in one of the 20th century's greatest medical breakthroughs. It wasn't until 1982, 17 years after his death, that Toronto historian Michael Bliss set the record straight on Collip's role in the dramatic dis-

covery of insulin. In his book *The Discovery of Insulin* . . . the team's achievement was clouded by a good deal of petty jealousy and backstabbing, mostly on Banting's part. When it came time to bask in the glory, Collip ended up in the shade." As an outsider, says Bliss, he didn't have "the powerful friends he needed when the struggle for recognition was going on." Afraid of being "closed out of the clinical trials" Banting secretly tried out a crude version of Collip's extract on human patients at Toronto General Hospital. The experiment was a "miserable failure" and "embarrassment." But "within a week of this failed experiment Collip struck gold. . . . He was able to isolate, or precipitate, the active principle in beef pancreas." On the night of his discovery, Collip wrote, "I experienced then and there all alone in the top floor of the old Pathology Building perhaps the greatest thrill which has ever been given me to realize." What followed was the now legendary confrontation between Collip and Banting, during which Collip, impatient with Banting's competitive attitude, threatened to keep the purification process to himself. Best later described the incident in a personal letter. "Banting was thoroughly angry and Collip was fortunate not be seriously hurt. I can remember restraining Banting with all the force at my command. . . . Collip's new extract was tested on 14-year-old Leonard Thompson, a severely diabetic patient. The results were unambiguously favorable. . . ." What had been a painful, devastating disease became manageable, and MacLeod and Banting were awarded the Nobel Prize for Medicine.

THE POLITICS OF RECOGNITION

"For the most part, history dropped Collip's name from the discovery of insulin, mainly because Banting was better able to orchestrate the politics of recognition from an eastern Canadian university. While MacLeod shared his portion of the Nobel Prize with Collip, the gesture did little to correct the public misconception of insulin as primarily Banting's discovery."

From article by Geoff McMaster, University of Alberta *Folio*. September 4, 1998.

Note 17.
Page 19, Paragraph 2
The company boasted a paid-in capital of only $4,250
Gary L. Nelson, Editor. *Pharmaceutical Company Histories, Volume One* "Ayerst Laboratories" p. 1–18 (Bismarck, N.D.: Woodbine Publishing, 1983.)
Wyeth-Ayerst Canada, Inc: A Canadian pharmaceutical success story
http://collections.ic.gc.ca/heirloom_series/volume 6

Note 18.
Page 19, Paragraph 3
although it did backfire with the contraceptive Norplant in the 1990s
"While Leiras has kept the price to developing countries at $23 per set, the cost in the United States was set much higher. Wyeth-Ayerst obtains its capsules from Leiras, repackages them with a few inexpensive items such as a plastic insert, and resells the kits for at least $350 wholesale. . . . However, as Norplant is particularly encouraged for low-income, single mothers, 50 to 60 percent of Norplant bills are paid by Medicaid—meaning that U.S. taxpayers are lavishly underwriting Wyeth-Ayerst. Under these circumstances how does the distributor justify its markup? At a hearing of the House Small Business Committee, company spokesman

Mark Deitch M.D. said the high price was intended to protect a marketing image, and to prevent middle-class women from shunning Norplant as a drug for the poor."

Barbara Seaman, *The Doctors' Case Against the Pill*, 25th Anniversary Updated Edition (Alameda California: Hunter House, 1995.)

Approved by the FDA in 1990, Norplant was withdrawn in 2002.

Note 19.
Page 20, Paragraph 1
It would have been interesting to have been a fly on the wall

J.B. Collip, co-discoverer of insulin in 1922, was at McGill University in 1929 when he was approached by W.J. McKenna of Ayerst, and Harrison to carry out studies on placental hormones. Their research led to the production in 1930 of Emmenin, the first of a series of research steps that led to the discovery of Premarin that Ayerst began marketing worldwide in 1941 and is exported to over 80 countries. The Canadian Medical Journal in 1930 contained three separate papers by Dr. Collip in which he step by step describes the isolation of Emmenin in its pure form from human placenta. Prepared and biologically standardized, according to Dr. Collip's technique (and with the approval of the Department of Biochemistry at McGill), Ayerst began to market Emmenin, based on the urine of Canadian women in the last trimester of pregnancy, called HPU for "human pregnancy urine."

From: http://collections.ic.gc.ca/heirloom_series/volume290

Note 20.
Page 20, Paragraph 2
scars from the insulin team

Eventually Drs. Gordon Grant and A. Stanley Cook at Ayerst readied Premarin for market.

Note 21.
Page 20, Paragraph 3
"Thus the laboratory embarked on a search for a new source"

Nelson, op. cit.

Note 22.
Page 21, Paragraph 4
The name changes of Premarin's parent corporation may be confusing

Nelson, op. cit.

Wyeth Timeline at www.Wyeth.com/about.timeline

Melody Petersen, "American Home Products is Changing Its Name to Wyeth," *New York Times*, March 11, 2002.

BUTENANDT SECTION

Note 23.
Page 22, Paragraph 2

Adolph Friedrich Johann Butenandt (b. March 24, 1903, Bremerhaven-Lehe, Ger. —d. Jan. 16, 1995, Munich) studied at Marburg and Gottingen, received his Ph.D. in 1927.

Arguably, he was the #1 sex hormone scientist of the twentieth century. After World War II, he shifted his interest to cancer research, and the active substances of insects. He remained in Germany during the war, and survived as one of that nation's most respected scientists, at home and abroad, for another 40 years. However, he may have had a double life. In 1984, Benno Muller-Hill, professor of genetics at the University of Cologne, was writing a book called *Murderous Science*, when he discovered that through a close associate, Dr. Gunther Hillman, Butenandt appeared to have connections to Nazi experiments. As the war was ending, Butenandt ordered many files and archival sources destroyed, but vigorously denied that he or the Kaiser Wilhelm Institutes had ever been involved in euthanasia programs, claims that no longer hold, as further research by Tubingen scholar Jurgen Peiffer shows. Scholars are presently investigating how much, if at all, Butenandt was involved with the Nazi experiments at Auschwitz, and why he might have been involved.

Note 24.
Page 24, Paragraph 3
Carl Djerassi e-mailed me

Born in Vienna and educated in the United States, Djerassi is a writer and professor of chemistry at Stanford University. Djerassi is author of over 1200 scientific articles, and winner of the National Medal of Science in 1973 for his work on the Pill. He is also the author of several nonfiction books, including *This Man's Pill: Reflections on the 50th Birthday of the Pill* (New York: Oxford University Press, 2001). Since reaching the age of 70, Djerassi has written five novels and three plays, all of them dealing with the personal and human conflicts of cutting-edge scientists. As a playwright himself, it is not surprising that in his e-mail of March 16, 2002, Djerassi made reference to Werner Heisenberg, Nobel-winning German physicist, whose complex relationship with Nazism is now well recognized, due to Michael Frayn's hit Broadway play, *Copenhagen.*

After comparing these two German Nobelists of the 1930s, the one in physics, the other in chemistry, Djerassi went on to say of Butenandt: "He died just a few years ago and was one of the most influential post-war German scientists in his capacity as President of the Max Planck Society. The last president of that society finally initiated a study of the Nazi involvement of the society and Butenandt is covered there."

Note 25.
Page 25, Paragraph 2
Butenandt was not anti-Semitic. He saved two Jewish scientists

Carl Neuberg (1877–1966). See Neuberg papers in American Philosophical Society in Philadelphia. www.amphilsoc.org "The Butenandt files in the Neuberg papers (1947–56 in German) document the strong bond between these two important biochemists."

Alfred Gottschalk (1894–1973). See Australian Academy of Science Biographical Memoirs. www.science.org.au/academy/memoirs Returning to Germany in 1963 "he was most warmly received (by) Professor Adolph Butenandt (who) offered him facilities and an honorarium."

But also see: Robert Proctor, *Adolph Butenandt* (1903–1995). Published in German. (Berlin-Presientenkcommission, 2000. 40 pp.)

Robert Proctor, *The Nazi War on Cancer*. New Jersey: Princeton University Press, 1999.

Note 26.
Page 26, Paragraph 1-2
"Why he would have turned a blind eye is not known." I'll tell you why.
Letter from Alison Abbott, *Nature* magazine correspondent, March 25, 2000.
Also see:
Alison Abbott, "German Science Begins to Cure Its Historical Amnesia," *Nature* magazine, Vol. 403, p. 474–475. (2000)
Alison Abbott and Quirin Schiermeier. "Deep Roots of Nazi Science Revealed," *Nature* magazine, Vol. 407, p. 823–824. (2000)

The clues to the Butenandt mystery begin with his curiously protective attitude toward Otmar Frieherr von Verschur. Of noble birth, and a eugenicist who wrote an influential 1930s textbook on racial cleansing, he was appointed, in 1942, to head the Kaiser Wilhelm Institute for Anthropology, Human Genetics, and Eugenics, located, like Butenandt's Kaiser Wilhelm Institute for Chemistry, in Berlin. Von Verschur had been an adviser to the Nazis on racial policies "at the highest level," as well as the supervisor of Dr. Josef Mengele in the notorious human experiments (including those where twins were deliberately infected with typhus or tuberculosis) that were performed at the Auschwitz concentration camp. Yet after the war, Butenandt, who was held in the highest esteem in the international galaxy of great scientists, vouched for von Verschur's integrity with such vigor that the latter, instead of being tried for war crimes, was appointed to a prestigious postwar professorship at a medical school. There must have been some who wondered why Butenandt would risk his own standing to protect a marginal scientist with obvious ties to the Third Reich. No one seems to have called Butenandt on it until 1984, when Benno Muller-Hill, professor of genetics at the University of Cologne, published a book called *Murderous Science* in which he revealed von Verschur's administrative role in the Auschwitz experiments, as well as the fact that the human blood samples were sent to Butenandt's Institute, for analysis by his close colleague and associate Gunther Hillmann (who would later be entrusted with destroying the records, at war's end). Butenandt and some of his influential former pupils threatened Muller-Hill with lawsuits, but he was too big a scientist for them to bring him down. (In 1964 Muller-Hill and Walter Gilbert had isolated the lactose repressor, the first example of a genetic control element, which won a Nobel prize for Gilbert in 1980.)

After the war, the Kaiser Wilhelm Society changed its name to the Max Planck Society, of which Butenandt was president from 1960–72.

At the present time, leaders of the Max Planck Society have vowed to "confront and discuss their past" in the Nazi era. Highly qualified historians have been appointed to investigate, but the effort is hampered by the fact that Butenandt's files are supposed to remain closed for 30 years after his death in 1995. Some exceptions are being made; but many records have been destroyed, so that the real facts may never be fully confirmed. Whether or not Butenandt was a Nazi, no one disputes that he was an ambitious, obsessive scientist and science administrator— as he had to be in order to accomplish all that he did. He also had to be extremely curious on the role his estrogens would play in contraception.

Suppose you were Butenandt, trying to protect your family and career in such a way that you could be sure to land on your feet after the war, win it or lose it. But then, suppose your patron Schering begged you to secure the future of ethinyl estradiol, on which the company had pinned so many hopes, by establishing the correct dose range. You wouldn't have to go near Auschwitz or attach your name to it in any way. You could silently "piggyback" on von Verschur/Mengele's investigations. Auschwitz doctors could perform examinations and collect your bloods and urine in the guise of their own research. If this is what happened, as I believe, it explains why Butenandt was determined to protect von Verschur from scrutiny. Had von Verschur been tried for war crimes, the Auschwitz chemical analyses performed in Butenandt's institute would likely have been revealed.

Note 27.
Page 27, Paragraph 3
Schering scientists Hans Herloff Inhoffen and Walter Hohlweg synthesized the aforementioned ethinyl estradiol, which remains the most popular estrogen used in birth control pills to this day

The Butenandt obituary that appeared in the *Boston Globe* on January 19, 1995, proclaimed that "His research helped lead to the invention of the birth control pill." Bostonians who believed all that magic happened exclusively at the labs of their own Dr. John Rock, of Harvard, and Dr. Gregory Pincus must have thought the AP in Germany was mistaken, as some readers of this book will also assume. If you are curious, you should be able to find the English version of detailed Schering company timelines on the Internet. For hormonal therapies try www.schering.de.eng/fertility. For general product histories try www.schering.de/eng/company/history. For all other information try http://www.schering.de/eng/index.html or a booklet called: "From a Chemist's Shop to a Multinational Enterprise Berlin (5th Ed)." Germany: Schering Aktiengesellschaft. 2001

You can also confirm at the patent office that at least three U.S. patents were issued to Schering for "estradiol-like" compounds before and during World War II. (The U.S. branch of Schering stayed open during World War II, although the U.S. Treasury Department seized it immediately after Pearl Harbor and ran it until 1952, when a group headed by Merrill Lynch bought it at auction. It was called Schering, Inc. until 1971 when U.S. Schering merged with Plough, Inc. Today, Berlex is the U.S. branch of the German Schering.)

See: Gary L. Nelson, Pharmaceutical Company Histories, Vol. 1, op cit., p. 141–155.

The three patents issued more than sixty years ago were:
2,096,744 Oct. 26, 1937
2,225,419 Dec. 17, 1940
2,361,847 Oct. 31, 1944

In the millennium edition of Dr. Richard Dickey's *Managing Contraceptive Pill Patients* (Dallas, Texas: Emis, Inc.), he lists 43 brands of combined contraceptives sold in the United States. Thirty-eight contain estradiol; only five contain mestranol, the product used in Searle's Enovid, the first U.S. birth control pill. Anovlar, Schering's first birth control pill, was introduced a few months later, in 1961. By 1949, after some wartime assistance from Adolph Butenandt, Schering had made ethinyl estradiol safe enough to place it on the commercial market.

It is the same component used today in the Schering/Berlex combination oral contraceptives, including newer ones such as Yasmin. As for brands from other manufacturers: "Ethinylestradiol has a specific chemical structure. So, when a product is said to contain ethinylestradiol, it contains the same chemical entity. It is possible that because manufacturing processes vary from company to company, there could be very slight differences . . . " explains Kimberly Schillace of Berlex.

For more specifics see Wolfgang Frobenius, A *Triumph of Scientific Research: the Development of Ethinylestradiol and Ethinyltestosterone, a Story of Challenges Overcome.* England: The Parthenon Publishing Group, 1990.

This report confirms that Hans Herloff Inhoffen worked as an assistant in Dodds's laboratory in London during 1935–36. "The Berlin Company made it possible for Inhoffen to spend time in England until 1936. During that period he worked at the Courtauld Institute of Biochemistry in London as an assistant to Charles Dodds. . . . These investigations were to lead, in 1938, to the preparation of stilbestrol . . . naturally of great interest to Schering as hormone manufacturers. In 1936 Inhoffen returned to Berlin and worked until 1945 as departmental manager in Schering's main laboratory." In the preface to Dr. Frobenius' book, Schering scientist Professor Friedmund Neumann asks why ethinyl estradiol was not introduced into the German market (under the name of Progynon C.) until 1949, 11 years after Hohlweg and Inhoffen published their paper. "Could it have been the fear of serious side effects?" he muses. He quotes Dr. Karl Junkmann (1897–1976), who took over as head of Schering research in 1945, indicating that "There was some evidence that this fear might have foundation, particularly since ethinyl estradiol had been overdosed by a factor of several hundred percent in the initial clinical studies" resulting in "almost uncontrollable bleeding during clinical trials at the Charite hospital" at the end of the 1930s.

Note 28.
Page 28, Paragraph 3

When I interviewed Dr. Jofen in 1976 she recalled that her work had already been ongoing for 20 years, which means that by the date of our last interview, September 10, 2002, she had been on this trail for close to half a century. In the 1960s and 70s, my editor and publisher Peter Wyden, born in Germany and a U.S Army intelligence officer there after the war, introduced me to Auschwitz survivors who independently confirmed what Jofen said. I included several pages on her study in my 1977 book *Women and the Crisis in Sex Hormones* (pp. 128–130). In our "25th anniversary" interview Dr. Jofen added information I hadn't heard before. She had tracked down several cooks who worked in the Auschwitz kitchens. Not only did they tell her the name of the liquid contraceptive, Salitrum, but they also mentioned that it came in barrels stamped I.G. Farben. She also found representatives of a group of 500 women who were moved from Auschwitz to another camp, Zaltswede, where there was nothing in the soup, and the menstruation of these women returned, Dr. Jofen said. For those too young to remember, I.G. Farben was a German cartel of five large corporations that dealt in all sorts of chemicals and had helped the government to ready Germany for an extended war. The name, I.G. Farben, was deceptively innocent, short for "Interessen Gemeinshaft Farbenindustrie" meaning "Community Interest of the Dye Industry." However, far from being limited to dye components, I.G. Farben, in association with lesser cartels and individual corporations (Schering rumored to be among them), was synthesizing all of the strategic raw materials that Germany lacked within its own borders, including fibers for every kind of fabric, oil, rubber, nitrates, poison gases, and rocket fuels.

Note 29.
Page 29, Paragraph 4
"We need a cage of ovulating females"

Lara V. Marks, *Sexual Chemistry: A History of the Contraceptive Pill* (New Haven and London: Yale University Press, 2001), p. 98.

Note 30.
Page 29, Paragraph 5
The following year Pincus . . . found his "cage of ovulating females"
See Gregory Pincus' correspondence at the Library of Congress on the Puerto Rican Pill trials 1956–59. Pincus was the opposite of Butenandt in that Pincus seems to have destroyed nothing, however embarrassing or less than ethical it might seem. One senses that he wanted to leave the world a true record of the scientific brinkmanship it takes to launch a new and daring drug.

Note 31.
Page 31, Paragraph 1
Strictly speaking, neither Searle's mestranol nor Schering's ethinyl estradiol were the first hormonal contraceptive. For example, both Carl Djerassi and Lara Marks write admiringly about an Austrian physiologist and social reformer, Ludwig Haberlandt, who devised progesterone based contraceptive called Infecundin that was registered in 1930. It was purchased by Gideon Richter, a Hungarian company interested in hormones, who renewed the commercial registration in 1940 and 1950. In 1966, Richter promoted Infecundin as the first Hungarian contraceptive pill. In addition, Marks informs us, "Infecundin or a similar substance called Profecundin, is also rumored to have been promoted in Germany during 1942." (Marks, *Sexual Chemistry*, page 48)

Whether we ever learn which specific hormones were dumped into the Auschwitz soup, there is no doubt that Butenandt had the knowledge, the opportunity, the motive, the access, and the means to execute estrogen trials at Auschwitz. Never was there a more captive "cage of ovulating females." If this is what happened, it readily explains why the Auschwitz bloods were sent to his institute, and why Butenandt was impelled, for his own protection, to "whitewash" Von Verschur after the war. The puzzle is why anyone would doubt that Butenandt, surely one of the most intensely-focused steroid chemists of all time, had the desire and the capacity to learn more about the manmade hormone products he, himself, had helped introduce into the world.

THE PANDORA'S BOX OF SIR CHARLIE DODDS

Note 32.
Page 32, Paragraph 3
distinguished chemists, including Edward Charles Dodds
Born October 13, 1899, Sir Edward Charles Dodds, M.D., Ph.D., M.V.O., was an international scientific statesman. Honorary Fellow of the Royal College of Pathologists, the Royal College of Physicians and Surgeons (Canada), and an Australian Postgraduate Fellow in Medicine, he held honorary degrees from universities at Cambridge (England), Glasgow, Bologna, and Chicago. He was president of the 4th International Congress of Endocrinology in 1968; chairman of the Scientific Advisory Committee, British Empire Cancer Campaign; the chairman of the Science Committee of the British Heart Foundation. He was an honorary member of the American Society of Clinical Pathologists; the American Association for Cancer Research; the New York Academy of Sciences; the Biological Society of Chile; the Society

of Chemical Industries of France; the Finnish Society of Medicine; the Royal Medical Academy of Barcelona; the Italian Chemical Society; the Danish Society of Internal Medicine; the Medical Society of Gothenburg (Sweden); and numerous others.

As a key transitional figure in the twentieth century marriage of pure science and applied technology, he served with organizations in England dealing with food additives and poisonous substances in agricultural use. He died in 1973.

See Robert Meyers, *D.E.S.: The Bitter Pill*. New York: Seaview/Putnam, 1983, pp. 30–31.

Note 33.
Page 33, Paragraph 2
name applied to these criminals: "the Devil's chemists"
    See
    The Intro to Crimes and Punishment of I.G. Farben
    http://home.earthlink.net/-x288files/I.G.intro.htm
    Human Sacrifice and Human Experimentation: Reflections at Nuremberg by Jay Katz.
Paper delivered in October 1996 at a conference commemorating the 50th anniversary of the Nazi Doctors Trial at Nuremberg. Yale School of Law Publications.
    Robert J. Lifton, *The Nazi Doctors*. New York: Basic Books, 2000.

Note 34.
Page 35, Paragraph 1
"Such products must stay in the public domain"
    Personal communication: Edward Charles Dodds to Barbara Seaman

Note 35.
Page 36, Paragraph 3
"We should always be humbled"
    Barbara Seaman, *The Doctors' Case Against the Pill*. New York: Wyden, 1969, p. 146

Note 36.
Page 37, Paragraph 3
Dodds sent Karnaky a study that he himself had performed
    British Medical Journal, September 10, 1938, pp. 557–9. Coauthored with A.S. Parkes and R.L. Noble, it was titled, "Interruption of Early Pregnancy by Means of Orally Active Oestrogens." This paper starts with a provocative statement. "It was found many years ago that the injection of oestrogenic extracts after mating interfered with the establishment of pregnancy." (One of the first people Dodds credits with this discovery is none other than Gregory Pincus, whose book *The Eggs of Mammals* was published in 1936.)

Dodds was of course extremely curious to compare stilbestrol with ethinyl estradiol, He was unable or unwilling to ask Schering for it directly, as "the ethinyl oestradiol was kindly supplied" by intermediaries, Dr. K. Miescher and Messrs. Ciba Limited. The study concluded that both substances, the British and the German, could interrupt an established pregnancy as well as preventing implantation of fertilized ova in both rabbits and rats, but ethinyl oestradiol was the more highly effective in interrupting established pregnancy in rabbits. Dodds concluded that Schering's brainchild was far stronger than his own. Inhoffen himself had calculated that ethinyl estradiol was seventeen times as active by mouth as oestradiol, while stilbestrol was about three times as active.

Note 37.
Page 38, Paragraph 1
The researcher, Dr. Michael Boris Shimkin

Born in Toms on the Russian frontier in 1912, his father worked on Trans-Siberian railway, his mother was a physician. He immigrated to the United States in 1921, became a citizen in 1928, died in 1989. Upon getting his M.D., Shimkin became one of the first research fellows of the National Cancer Institute, which was then located at Harvard. A leading cancer researcher of his generation, he published over 300 articles representing clinical and laboratory research on tumors in mice, the effects of carcinogens, chemotherapies and analyses of cancer statistics. He was the editor of the journal *Cancer Research*, scientific editor of the *Journal of the National Cancer Institute*, and author of two books on the history of the study of cancer. He held the following positions: Chief of Biometry and Epidemiology Branch of National Cancer Institute, Vice President for Research at Temple University Health Science Center, Professor of Community Medicine and Oncology at the University of California San Diego, and President of the American Association for Cancer Research.

From: the Michael B. Shimkin papers at the University of California, San Diego.

Note 38.
Page 38, Paragraph 3
The Shimkin-Grady paper was far from the only warning

The following among many others were published in respected journals:

Geshicter, as noted, in *Radiology* in 1939; Shimkin and Grady in *Journal of the National Cancer Institute* in October, 1940; Greene, Burrill, and Ivy in the *American Journal of Anatomy and Science* and other publications in 1939–40; and Edgar Allen and W.U. Gardner in *Cancer Research* in April 1941.

Note 39.
Page 39, Paragraph 2
In 1976, after the discovery of the tragedies in some

Summary of DES effects can be found on the DES Action website:
http://www.DESAction.org

DES Action was founded and is run by and for afflicted families. Mother and daughter Pat and Nora Cody, who, having devoted themselves to these matters for a quarter of a century, are always up to date on the research and treatments, maintain this site. Some DES-exposed mothers and daughters, including the late Congresswoman Patsy Mink, have brought successful lawsuits.

DES (diethylstilbestrol) is a synthetic estrogen drug that was given to millions of pregnant women primarily from 1938–1971. Use of DES during pregnancy was thought to prevent miscarriage and ensure a healthy pregnancy. DES did not work, and women who took DES and the children they carried are at risk for certain health problems and may need special care.

Breast cancer: Women who took DES have a somewhat higher risk for breast cancer. They should pay particular attention to their breast care: practice monthly breast self-exam, have annual clinical breast exams and mammography.

Cancer: All DES daughters (women whose mothers took DES while pregnant with them) have a risk of about 1 in 1,000 for a rare cancer of the vagina or cervix called clear cell adenocarcinoma.

Infertility: DES Daughters have an increased risk for infertility.

Pregnancy Problems: DES Daughters have a higher risk for ectopic pregnancy, miscarriage, and pre-term labor and delivery.

Structural Changes in Reproductive Organs: DES daughters have an increased incidence of structural changes in their reproductive organs.

Some DES sons face problems with their genital organs.

Note 40.
Page 39, Paragraph 2
I asked the Smiths if they had been aware of any of this research
Barbara Seaman and Gideon Seaman, M.D., *Women and the Crisis in Sex Hormones.* op. cit., p. 6–10.

Note 41.
Page 43, Paragraph 1
In a bizarre twist, the Nobel Prize for a DES application
Charles Brenton Huggins (b. Sept. 22, 1901, Halifax, Nova Scotia, Canada. d. January 12, 1997, Chicago, Ill.) was a specialist in the male urological and genital tract. He joined the faculty at the University of Chicago in 1927. In the early 1940s he found that he could retard the growth of prostate cancer by blocking the action of the patient's male hormones with doses of the female hormone estrogen.

Note 42.
Page 45, Paragraph 5
FDA officially approved the use of stilbestrol
For further information on the successful campaign for approval of DES in 1941, see the chapter "Government Approval and the Marketing of DES" in Robert Meyers, *D.E.S.: The Bitter Pill*, op. cit., pp. 56–72. On p. 63 Meyers explains that DES was "officially approved by the FDA for use in four types of treatment: gonorrheal vaginitis, menopausal symptoms, senile vaginitis, and to prevent lactation in women who had recently given birth. . . . Once it was approved for limited purposes the law permitted it to be used by physicians for other purposes, in an experimental capacity." "It is at this point," Meyers continues, immediately after the FDA's initial approval of DES for use with menopausal women, that the interest in using DES to prevent miscarriages accelerated. It was used first by Karl John Karnaky in Houston with results published in 1942, then with Priscilla White and the Smiths' diabetic patients in Boston, then in the early trials conducted by George and Olive Smith, published in 1946. DES was approved for use in preventing miscarriages in 1947, although it had been widely used on what was called an experimental basis before that. There was far less intense lobbying in order to get this additional approval, as far as can be gleaned from the public record.

On a Personal Note: The Most Heartbreaking Collection.
In 1979, Joyce Bichler, a beautiful young New York woman, was the first DES daughter who won damages for the radical cancer surgery that saved her life but left her unable to ever

bear children. I testified at her trial that I believed the drug companies could have, should have, *and quite possibly did* know that this drug might cause cancer in offspring due to the previous animal research before it was even cleared for marketing in 1941. Lilly certainly knew about the intersexuality as evidenced in papers submitted to the FDA on 5-23-1940, and withdrawn on 11-11-1940 when they learned that the FDA had decided to turn down the marketing applications. These original papers seem to me to paint a strikingly different picture from those organized the following year by the Small Committee and Carson P. Frailey. A 1940 paper, called The Toxicity of Stilbestrol, by Drs. K.K. Chen and P.N. Harris of the Lilly Research Laboratories was learned, thorough, and alarming to those who take animal studies to heart . . . "Confirmation of Dodds' work has come from various sources (10) (11) (12) (13) (14) (15) (16) . . . While Houverswyn, Folley, and Gardner showed mammary growth of male mice after stilbestrol, Lacassagne produced mammary adenocarcinoma in the same sex of a susceptible strain. As with estradiol, intersexuality occurred in male rats, mice or chickens when stilbestrol was administered. . . . Stilbestrol reduced milk production in animals, caused abortion in cows."

CHAPTER 3: HOW HAS PREMARIN FARED IN THE UNITED STATES, AND WHO WAS ROBERT WILSON?

Note 43.
Page 47, Paragraph 1
"an enthusiastic man, a man with a vision"
  Gary L. Nelson, ed. *Pharmaceutical Company Histories*. Volume 1. op. cit., p. 4

Note 44.
Page 48, Paragraph 1
associated with estrogen, including Premarin, in mice, rats, rabbits, hamsters
  Interview with Dr. Roy Hertz by Dr. Roald Grant, editor of *CA*, a journal published by the American Cancer Society.
  Barbara Seaman, *The Doctors' Case Against the Pill*, 1969, op. cit., pp. 163–165

Note 45.
Page 48, Paragraph 2
After the first year on Premarin, one woman in ten
  Barbara Seaman interviews with Diana Petitti, M.D., April 2002
  Barbara Seaman and Gideon Seaman, M.D., *Women and the Crisis in Sex Hormones*, op. cit., ch29 "ERT and Cancer" pp. 401–407
  "Endometrial Cancer" by Linda S. Cook and Noel S. Weiss, pp. 916–931 in *Women and Health*, Marlene B. Goldman and Maureen C. Hatch, Editors, San Diego, Ca: Academic Press, 2000

Note 46.
Page 49, Paragraph 1
Harry Loynd, who, like McKenna
  Thomas Maeder, *Adverse Reactions*. New York: William Morrow, 1994.

Note 47.
Page 49, Paragraph 2
depicts a harpy who obviously has just done something awful . . .
   Barbara Seaman and Gideon Seaman, M.D., *Women and the Crisis in Sex Hormones.*
op. cit., p. 342

Notes 48, 49, 50.
Pages 52–53
   Robert Wilson: op. cit., p. 352
   David Reuben: op. cit., p. 374
   Robert Wilson and FDA: op. cit., p. 351–352

Note 51.
Page 53, Paragraph 1
Dr. Jay S. Cohen scolded the company
   Jay S. Cohen, "Do Standard Doses of Frequently Prescribed Drugs Cause Preventable Adverse Effects in Women?" *The Journal of the American Medical Women's Association* *(JAMWA).* Spring 2002.

Note 52.
Page 53
   BRS interviews with Dr. Robert Wilson, Dr. J. Richard Crout, and Mallon de Santis.
   Barbara Seaman and Gideon Seaman, M.D., *Women and the Crisis in Sex Hormones.*

Note 53.
Page 54, Paragraph 4
David Sackett . . . spoke for me
   David Sackett, "The Arrogance of Preventive Medicine," *CMAJ (Canadian Medical Association Journal).* August 20, 2002.

Note 54.
Page 55, Paragraph 3
Thanks to my late father
   Interviews and correspondence BRS and Ron Wilson:
   September 2002, most concentrated September 8 and 9:
   father committed suicide   9/9/02 7:43 am
   father always drank   9/9/02 11:13 am
   father born April 18, 1895 at Vale House, Newchurch,
   Rastenstall, England. Became U.S. citizen June 18,
   1940. Died August 21, 1981   9/9/02 7:29 pm
   death of Thelma Amelia Wilson, and the husband who told
   her Premarin was safe   9/8/02 4:56 pm

Note 55.
Page 59, Paragraph 3
She goes to a health club three times a week, spends a half hour on a bike
   "Old, Sharp, and Still Working," by Shirley Camper Soman in NYPC BYTES at www.nypc.org

Note 56.
Page 59, Paragraph 3
How did Sandra Gorney legitimize and iconize
   Barbara Seaman and Gideon Seaman, M.D., *Women and the Crisis in Sex Hormones,* op. cit., pp. 353–4.
   Another talented medical writer, working directly for Ayerst in this period, was Lois Gaeta. She edited a magazine for the Ayerst sales force called *Scoreboard.* The cover story in the January 1970 issue was titled "The Flowering of Premarin in Japan." The strategy for getting doctors to use Premarin was to introduce it to them for treating heavy uterine bleeding (FDA approved, but rarely used). "Our job was to make it a standard for hemorrhagic indications throughout the country while 'laying the groundwork' for gradually influencing doctors and women to think of menopause as an estrogen deficiency disease." The company retained "professor-physicians" to present papers on Premarin. Mailings to "ladies' societies" offered them guest lecturers. Posters were placed in gynecological outpatient departments and brochures in physicians' waiting rooms. "There was also the insertion of physician-written ERT articles in favored ladies' journals."

CHAPTER 4: A DARING PROJECT TO KEEP WOMEN YOUNG

Note 57.
Page 61, Paragraph 1
two major papers on hot flashes
   L.F. Hawkinson, "The menopausal syndrome: one thousand consecutive patients with estrogen," *Journal of the American Medical Association* 11; 390–393 (1938)
   Weisbader and Kurzork, "The menopause: a consideration of the symptoms, etiology and treatment by means of estrogens," *Endocrinology* 23; 32–38 (1938)

Note 58
Page 62, Paragraph 3.
Dr. Robert Benjamin Greenblatt graduated
   Dr. Robert Benjamin Greenblatt, known as "Bob" (b. Oct 12, 1906 in Montreal, Canada. d. September 27, 1987 in Augusta, Georgia), was an influential researcher and medical educator on long-term hormone use and infertility treatments. He developed implants as a system of delivery, including a regimen for estradiol pellet implantation that pointed the way to long-acting hormonal birth control. With Dr. Virendra Mahesh, he discovered source of polycystic ovary syndrome. He also did pioneering research on antibiotics in venereal disease. He was a public health hero, a Navy war hero in WWII, prolific author and lecturer, Professor, Medical College of Georgia (1935–74), Professor and Chairman of the Department of

Endocrinology (1946–72), Professor Emeritus of Endocrinology (1974–87). Institute Robert B. Greenblatt, Bordeaux, France in 1985, and Medical College of Georgia Library in 1988 were named for him.

Note 59.
Page 63, Paragraph 2
But Greenblatt never stopped obsessing over hormones
    Greenblatt, R.B, *J. Am. Med. Assoc.* 121:17.1943
    Greenblatt, R.B. J. Editorial, "Hormone Factors in Libido," *Journal of Clinical Endocrinology*. Editorial, May 1943, pp. 305–306

Note 60.
Page 64, Paragraph 5
    Virendra B. Mahesh was born in Khanki, Punjab, India (now Pakistan) on April 25, 1932, received his first Ph.D. (organic chemistry) at Delhi University and his second (biological sciences) at Oxford. While there he developed new methods for measuring hormones in blood and urine, and famously treated twin sisters of whom "one developed severe hirsutism after an emotional crisis while the other was normal." In 1958 he accepted a research fellowship at Yale. Greenblatt, who "had a very large number of patients with hirsutism and virilism," spirited Mahesh away from New Haven to join his Augusta research group "as an equal partner in the discovery of new knowledge." The outcome was that, together, Mahesh and Greenblatt became the world authorities on polycystic ovaries. At 70, Mahesh is a Regents Professor and Chairman Emeritus, Dept. of Physiology and Endocrinology, Medical College of Georgia and Editor in Chief, *Biology of Reproduction*.
    BRS correspondence or interviews with Virendra Mahesh: 2/21/02, 3/1/02, 3/13/02, 3/15/02, 10/30/02, 11/22/02, 12/10/02.

Note 61.
Page 65, Paragraph 1
Greenblatt also enlisted help from his relatives
    BRS interview with Edward Greenblatt, August 20, 2002.
    BRS interview with Debbie Greenblatt-Neese, November 2, 2002.

Note 62.
Page 68, Paragraph 1
Greenblatt wrote a popular manual called Office Endocrinology . . .
    Robert B. Greenblatt, *Office Endocrinology*. Springfield, Ill. Charles C. Thomas, 4 Editions, 1941–52.

Note 63.
Page 69, Paragraph 3
he acknowledged that this cancer could be avoided
    The conflict and dilemma for doctors is that many women who feel good on estrogen alone complain that the addition of progestins makes them moody, depressed, and nervous. It may be for this reason, and because most of their members believed in the value of "keeping her on Premarin" that the American College of Obstetricians and Gynecologists (ACOG)

was hesitant to acknowledge the magnitude of the cancer risk for women who have uteruses but prefer to take estrogen alone. In FDA's "Labeling Guidance for Estrogen Drug Products" issued in February 1990, the agency stated that "Endometrial cancer is especially increased with long term use, with increased risks of 15 to 24 fold (!) for five to ten years or more." This statistic notwithstanding, in April 1992, ACOG issued Technical Bulletin #166 in which it recklessly stated "Estrogen-only therapy can be given, but endometrial biopsy should be performed prior to the initiation of therapy and annually thereafter." In 1991, the National Women's Health Network (NWHN) was troubled to learn the original design for the hormone studies included an arm where volunteers with intact uteruses would be given estrogen alone. On December 13, 1991 NWHN sent a protest letter to Dr. Bernadine Healy: "It is not ethical for the government to randomize women to a treatment with an established and unnecessary risk." Overriding the cautionary views of FDA, as well as NWHN and other women's health organizations that represent patients, Healy decided to follow the policies of ACOG. However, on November 17, 1994, a report from a clinical trial called PEPI (Postmenopausal Estrogen/Progestin Interventions) revealed very high rates of endometrial overgrowths, even though the study, with 875 volunteers, lasted only 3 years. The WHI investigators set up an Ad Hoc Group "to evaluate the PEPI findings and to propose the recommendations for modifying the WHI trial if needed." Based on the PEPI findings, the group concluded that after five years "only a small number of the WHI women with a uterus would still be on unopposed estrogen treatment. MOST of them would have developed overgrowths at best, and, at worst, cancers." On January 10, 1995 the Ad Hoc Group recommended "unopposed estrogen no longer be administered to women with a uterus." The women who have previously been assigned to unopposed estrogen will be changed to estrogen/progestin therapy only after a modified consent form is approved. A newsletter explaining these changes was mailed to all participants by January 14, 1995, and to the women's health advocates who had signed the protest letter to Dr. Healy. Dr. Loretta P. Finnegan, then the Director of the WHI, added a personal note to the women who'd tried to stop this folly in the first place inviting them to call her if they had any questions. A little known fact is that an arm of the WHI (estrogen only for women with uteruses) was halted in January 1995. The reason was that the WHI scientists made the mistake of trusting ACOG's protocol over the more conservative and cautious findings of the FDA, and women's health groups whose track record of protesting unproven medical treatments has panned out at almost 100%. Thus the halting of the Prempro arm in 2002 was not the first such incident.

See: Charles Mann, "Women's Health Research Blossoms." *Science Magazine*, Vol. 269, August 11, 1995, pp. 766–770

Endometrial cancer has increased in recent years some say, in part, because of the increase in obesity, but we can be sure that if women who quit Prempro go back on estrogen alone, endometrial cancer will zoom.

CHAPTER 5: CRAZY PEOPLE IN AMERICA

Note 64.
Page 73, Paragraph 1
There was hardly a day in 1938

Some were crackpots or dreamers but many were respectable or even eminent. For example, Priscilla White, M.D., founder of the Joslin Pregnancy Clinic for Diabetics in

Boston, was a leading researcher in the management of diabetic pregnancy. In 1936 and 1937, Dr. White treated pregnant diabetics experimentally with Butenandt's products prolutun and progynon, but no sooner did Dodds publish his formula than she switched to stilbestrol. In 1979 she explained her reasons in an affidavit: " . . . Between 1936 and 1938 I began treating pregnant diabetics with prolutin and progynon. . . . Because this treatment was administered usually at home daily by family members in the form of intramuscular injections, it ran the risk of infection which attends any therapy of repeated injection. Furthermore it was prohibitively expensive.

"When stilbestrol became available in 1938, I began using it for the treatment of pregnant diabetics. On the basis of my clinical experience, I devised a dosage schedule commencing early in pregnancy and continuing until delivery."

Source: DES Action Archive, Courtesy of Pat Cody.

Note 65.
Page 73, Paragraph 1
this Texas fellow, Karl John Karnaky,

In 1974, three years after the rare DES-daughter cancers were discovered and described, Karnaky distributed a bizarre flyer from his Research Foundation and Institute at 2164 Addison in Houston, Texas. He claimed that in 36 years of extensive stilbestrol use there had been not a single instance of vaginal adenosis or cancer in his practice. Instead he blamed "masturbation" for adenosis, a rare glandular structure in the vagina, reported as characteristic of daughters' exposed to diesthylstibestrol in the womb. He wrote in his flyer:

"OVER SEXUAL STIMULATED—as seen in the present day SEXUAL CRAZE— these are the young girls who almost daily stick something (or finger or fingers) into their vagina—appearing to be enjoying it with trauma to vaginal walls and cervix with . . . producing . . . of adenosis." Dr. Karnaky's flyer included a testimonial from a nun, Sister Edith, R.R.A., Director of the Medical Records at St. Joseph's

Source: DES Action Archive, Courtesy of Pat Cody

Note 66.
Page 74, Paragraph 2
Kennedy invited Cowan to testify at his Senate hearing

"The Cowan Study" Barbara Seaman and Gideon Seaman, M.D., *Women and the Crisis in Sex Hormones,* op. cit., p. 51–53.

Note 67.
Page 75, Paragraph 1
With his colleagues Patricia Smith and Anna Richardson,

F. Albright, P. Smith, and R. Richardson, "Postmenopausal osteoporosis and its clinical features." *Journal of the American Medical Association* 117:2473–2476.

Note 68.
Page 76, Paragraph 1
not be until a 1984 landmark Consensus Conference

NIH Consensus Development Statement on Osteoporosis, April 2–4 1984 Volume 5, No. 3.U.S. Department of Health and Human Services, National Institutes of Health, Office of Medical Applications of Research, Bethesda, Md 20205 Chairman of Consensus Panel, William A. Peck, M.D., Washington University School of Medicine.

Note 69.
Page 76, Paragraph 2
The Medical Letter 15:6–8 (1973)

Note 70.
Page 77, Paragraph 1
Harry Genant changed all that
Harry K. Genant was born in Freeport, Ill., in 1942. He attended the University of Illinois and Northwestern, served his internship at Johns Hopkins, residency at University of Chicago. In 1975 he joined faculty at University of California at San Francisco where he is a Professor in several departments and Executive Director of the Osteoporosis and Arthritis Research Group. His paper confirming Albright's theories appeared in *Ann Intern Med* 97:699–705, 1982.

Note 71.
Page 77, Paragraph 2
Something gets lost in translation
Patient advocacy groups such as Breast Cancer Action in San Francisco refer to such tactics as "science by press release." In its BCA e-newsletter for December, 2002, there was an item called "ERT and BC," another example of science by press release. The study claims "menopausal women who receive estrogen replacement therapy after being successfully treated for localized breast cancer have disease-free survival rates comparable to their counterparts who do not receive ERT. In other words, estrogen replacement therapy is supposedly safe for women who have had breast cancer and are currently free of the disease.—A closer look suggests that women . . . should be very cautious before taking estrogen based on this study. The study only looked at women whose breast cancer was estrogen receptor negative."
This is a similar to the misrepresentations of Genant's study. Most breast cancers are *estrogen receptive*, but those that are not—as the very name conveys—are less likely to grow when exposed to estrogen. "Science by press release" is a highly effective way of confusing patients (as well as doctors who are failing to check out original sources) into believing that successful drug treatments apply to a larger population pool than the actual study justifies.

Note 72.
Page 78, Paragraph 2
It was chaired by Dr. William Peck, professor (and later dean)
On January 28, 2000, when the *St. Louis Business Journal* ran its In Depth story: "100 Leaders for the Millennium," Dr. Peck, a prominent civic figure in St. Louis, was included: "Dr. William Peck, Executive vice chancellor for medical affairs and dean of the School of Medicine, Washington University. As dean since 1989 and executive vice chancellor for medical affairs since 1993, Dr. William Peck has protected and promoted the interests of Washington University's medical school, widely regarded as the University's crown jewel. Currently he is helping direct the largest building boom in the medical center's history. At age 66, the big questions are, when will Peck turn over the reins and who will be his successor?"

Who indeed? Dr. Peck is a premier example of a savvy medical educator and "player" in local and national health care politics, who helped lead the way to a growing presence of industry in medical school research, not only at his own institution but everywhere. When Washington University announced the formation of a search committee to choose his successor, their news release boasted: "Bill Peck is without a doubt one of the most effective leaders in the history of American Medical Education. . . . Total research funding to the Washington University School of Medicine in 2000−01 was more than $326 million from governmental and private sources." Thus, Peck is a superstar among medical school deans. Peck has recently completed terms as chair of the Association of American Medical Colleges (AAMC) and Chair of the AAMC Council of Deans. William Arno Peck was born in New Britain, Conn. September 28, 1933. He received his B.A. from Harvard and his M.D. from the University of Rochester. A decade after his 1984 Consensus Conference, I asked Dr. Peck what he thought of the results. He replied: "It brought recognition that osteoporosis is a major public health problem, it catapulted it into the public eye." In 1987 Peck chaired or cochaired two further influential meetings on osteoporosis one, again, for NIH and the other for FDA. However, in terms of our story, the most striking feature of his bio is that in 1985, the year following his successful Consensus Conference, Peck became Founding President of the National Osteoporosis Foundation, a position he held until 1990. The Osteoporosis Foundation does some excellent educational work but it is supported by industry, which most likely required Peck to fundraise. Bearing this in mind, many of the public positions he held would have posed potential conflicts of interest. Peck is a learned authority on the study of bone cell function and the causes of osteoporosis. He has written more than 100 scientific publications on bone and mineral metabolism, and has served as editor or advisor to various related journals and textbooks. He has also chaired the endocrine and metabolism FDA Advisory Committee, NIH study sections, and has served as president of the American Society for Bone and Mineral Research.

Peck is also a member of the Board on Health Sciences Policy of the National Academies/ Institute of Medicine. "Of particular concern" to this influential body "are the public and private policies and institutional arrangements that shape the way in which these sciences are structured, funded and coordinated." Adding one "power point" to another, Peck has wielded immeasurable influence on what osteoporosis research will be published or discarded, what drugs in the field will be approved for which indications, what standards medical schools will require in their research contracts with industry. (In some, the founder can block publication of an unfriendly research outcome, in others not.) I had an uncomfortable interview with Peck in the early 1990s when I asked him if it was true that some bone densitometry equipment was not reliable. He said that one brand was very good, but he could not tell me which because he was a director of the company. In 1998 Dr. Peck was listed in *Who's Who in America*, as a director of the following companies: Angelica Corp., Boatman's Trust Co., Allied Healthcare Products, Hologic, and Reinsurance Group of America. Hologic is a maker of equipment for osteoporosis detection. On December 3, 2002 Peck was reported to have participated in "Insider Trading" on Angelica stock on 5/29/2002, 8/23/2001, and 5/30/2001 (See Edgar Online http://biz.yahoo.com/t/A/AGL.html. According to Forbes, Angelica provides textile rental and laundry services to healthcare and other institutions and operates a chain of retail stores for nurses and other healthcare professionals.) RiverVest, a Capital Venture firm that has raided 89 million to invest in life science firms, also lists William Peck as a scientific advisor. Their posting states that he is also a member of the Scientific Advisory Committee of Johnson and Johnson, which manufactures hormone products.

Dr. Peck has been a key figure not only in educating the public on osteoporosis prevention through bone scanning and pharmacological treatment, but also in changing the atmosphere of medical education into one that includes a great deal of partnering with industry.

Note 73.

Page 78, Paragraph 2

a fiasco in which, according to Dr. Suzanne Parisian

Personal interviews and correspondence, June 1991, November, December 1991.

Also, see her extraordinary book *FDA Inside and Out,* which maps the machinery and the workings of this agency from a candid insider perspective.

S. Parisian, M.D. *FDA Inside and Out.* Front Royal, Va.: Fast Horse Press, 2001

Dr. Parisian, founder of Medical Device Assistance, Inc., a regulatory and medical consulting firm, is former Chief Medical Officer at FDA's Office of Device Evaluation.

Note 74.

Page 83, Paragraph 1

If Dodds was reluctant to have DES prescribed casually, he nonetheless felt empathy for women with "disturbing symptoms" that were "so often present in the menopause." He suggested: "It is found that if oestrogens are administered to the patient in decreasing amounts over period of about one year the symptoms are suppressed during the course of the therapy and do not recur when it is finally discontinued."

CHAPTER 6: CENSORSHIP

Note 75.

Page 85, Paragraph 1

Letter from Dr. Lila Wallis, Oct. 14, 2002

Note 76.

Page 86, Paragraph 1

How about substituting Dr. X

There is a back-story to this. On June 15, 1990, Dr. Barrett Connor was brought to the FDA by Wyeth-Ayerst to speak at the meeting being held to decide if Premarin would be approved for heart disease prevention. She was a bit embarrassed. The transcript shows that she said, "I would like you to know that I have not accepted undue remuneration. I came here coach class."

She had recently finished a 10-clinic lipid research study. She showed a series of slides which made it clear that *at baseline* "the women who were taking estrogen were significantly thinner, and I think that has been universally shown—women who get estrogen are thinner and had significantly better, that is to say higher levels of HDK than women not using estrogen, so they were healthier" (to start with). . . . "They were also less likely to smoke. . . . Women who got estrogen were much more likely to have completed high school. . . . the women who have received estrogen have been of a higher social class and thinner, at least two important variables which might determine their success." Dr. Barrett-Connor concluded, "I must say I am very torn." She thought perhaps the estrogen *was* good for the heart, and yet, it seemed that the women who took it were healthier to start with. Wyeth-Ayerst seemed not to be sure they got their money's worth by flying her in from California, even on coach.

From: Rockville, Maryland: Transcript of Proceedings Food and Drug Administration, Fertility and Maternal Health Drugs Advisory Committee.

Note 77.

Page 86, Paragraph 2

Sandra Coney, *The Menopause Industry, How the Medical Establishment Exploits Women.* Alameda, California: Hunter House, 1994.

Note 78.

Page 87, Paragraph 1

Alfred Goodman Gilman et al, *The Phamacological Basis of Therapeutics, 8th Edition.* New York: Pergamon Press, 1990.

Note 79.

Page 88, Paragraph 2

"Medical Dispatches: The Estrogen Question, How wrong is Dr. Susan Love?," *The New Yorker,* June 17, 1997.

Note 80.

Page 88, Paragraph 4

I was also flabbergasted when

The encounter took place at the 46th Annual Clinical Meeting of ACOG, on May 9–13, 1998 in New Orleans, Louisiana:

"Our session was on Tuesday May 12 and was termed the 4th Scientific Session: Controversies in Hormone Replacement Therapy."

Note 81.

Page 89, Paragraph 2

Alicia Mundy, *Dispensing with the Truth, The Victims, the Drug Companies, and the Dramatic Story Behind the Battle over Fen-Phen.* New York: St. Martin's Press, 2001.

Also see Forbes Alerts such as

9.27.02 Wyeth warns may need more reserves for diet litigation

Wyeth lowers profit view, raises Fen-Phen reserve

9.30.02 Research Alert-Morgan cuts Wyeth price target

10.03.02 Test-Fitch affirms Wyeth ratings

"The Negative Rating outlook reflects near-to-intermediate term risks that the company may experience further erosion in revenues from the Premarin product franchise and continue manufacturing issue, and the uncertainty with regard to the total cost of the diet drug litigation."

Note 82.

Page 90, Paragraph 2

Among the first to check them out was Judith Raphael Kletter

From correspondence with Judith Raphael Kletter 9.04.02 and 10.07.02

Note 83.

Page 94, Paragraph 3

"Prescription Drug Information. What is useful for the patient?" February 14–15, 1996, Doubletree Hotel, Rockville, Md.

FDA/Sponsored by U.S. Food and Drug Administration Office of External Affairs.

Note 84.

Page 96, Paragraph 9

Some reporters at the FDA workshop

"Pharmacists, doctors oppose rule to attach warnings to risky drugs," Lauran Neergaard, Associated Press, 2/27/96: *Hartford Courant* and various papers.

"Safety RX: Our View: The FDA wants consumers to have more information on drugs. What took them so long?" *USA Today* 2/19/96

Note 85.

Page 97, Paragraph 2

The Pill

The Doctors' Case Against the Pill 25th Anniversary Edition, reviewed by Carl J. Levinson M.D., Stanford University

Books Journals New Media *JAMA* July 10, 1996, vol 276, No 2, p. 166

Also see Letters; May 13, 1998, pp. 1443–44 "The Pill-25 Years Ago and Today"

Also see Sidney Wolfe, M.D., et al, "Questionable Doctors, Disciplined by State and Federal Governments 2000 Editions /Public Citizen Health Research Group"

California Edition CA-p. 194 Levinson, Carl J. license number 00G40673, Disciplined by California on January 28, 1996 Offense: Overprescribing or Misprescribing Drugs

New York Edition NY-p218 license number074197, Disciplined by New York on January 3, 1997.

Note 86.

Page 100, Paragraph 2

Documents available from The Food and Drug Archive Library IHS Health Information (1-800-525-5539)

CHAPTER 7: MADELINE GRAY

Note 87.

Page 110, Paragraph 2

Gray liked to update her subtitles with her various editions. For example, her first edition, published in 1951, is subtitled "What to do about the menopause." Her 1967 edition (the third, with 1958 in between) is subtitled "The Menopause Without Fear." The titles of her previous books were: *How to Cook for Profit; How to be a Success in the Restaurant Business;* and *The Bright Idea Book.*

Note 88.
Page 113, Paragraph 5
MalePractice
    Robert S. Mendelsohn, M.D., *MalePractice: How Doctors Manipulate Women*, Chicago: Contemporary Books, 1981.

Note 89.
Page 114, Paragraph 2
    Guttmacher's articles were coauthored with Ray E. Trussel and Mildred A. Morehead of the Columbia University School of Public Health. The Teamsters Union Joint Council 16 had requested them, and the research performed in the late 1950s and early 1960s.

Note 90.
Page 117, Paragraph 4
    "Estrogenic Hormones in the Genesis of Tumors and Cancers" by Edgar Allen, *Endocrinology*, June 1942.
    Presented with illustrations as the Presidential Address at the twenty-sixth annual meeting of the Association for the Study of Internal Secretions at Atlantic City, June 8, 1942. This paper contains a reference list of 77 articles bearing on estrogen and cancer, some of them published as early as 1938.
    Also, to get the flavor of deep concern about estrogen in that era, see the *Journal of the American Medical Association*, December 23, 1939; Council on Pharmacy and Chemistry by Ephraim Shorr, Frank H. Robinson and George N. Pananicolau and further articles and editorials. pp. 2312–2324.
    The concern was international as expressed in the reports from A. Lacassagne, at l'Institut Pasteur.

CHAPTER 8: POISON BY PRESCRIPTION

Note 91.
Page 119, Paragraph 3
Dr. Elizabeth Siegel Watkins, a Harvard-trained historian,
    Elizabeth Siegel Watkins, *On the Pill: A Social History of Oral Contraceptives, 1950–1970*, Baltimore: The Johns Hopkins University Press. 1998.

Note 92.
Page 120, Paragraph 3
Much less recognized . . . was Charlie Dodds's misbegotten diethystilbetrol
    Barbara Seaman and Gideon Seaman, M.D., *Women and the Crisis in Sex Hormones*, op. cit., p. 1–62.

Note 93.
Page 122, Paragraph 1
who would eventually become the father of Earth Day
    In 1995, Gaylord Nelson was awarded the Medal of Freedom, our nation's highest civilian honor. President Clinton said, "As the father of Earth Day he is the grandfather of all

that grew out of that event, the Environmental Protection Act, The Clean Air Act, the Safe Drinking Water Act." In 1980 after three remarkable terms in the Senate, Nelson was narrowly defeated in the Ronald Reagan landslide by only 59,000 votes out of more than 2.1 million. However he quit politics to choose a more retiring life as Director of the Wilderness Society.

Note 94.
Page 124, Paragraph 2
Wyeth is trying to take up the slack with aggressive promotion
Paul Glade, "From the Maker of Effexor: Campus Forums on Depression." *Wall Street Journal,* October 10, 2002

Note 95.
Page 124, Paragraph 3
See Exhibits, page 5921, Hearings Before the Subcommittee on Monopoly/Select Committe on Small Business United States Senate Ninety First Congress Second Session on Present Status of the Competition in the Pharmaceutical Industry Part 15, January 14, 21, 22 and 23, 1970 Oral Contraceptives (Volume 1) US Government Printing Office, Washington 1970.
Three Books, Parts 15, 16 and 17, also identified as Volumes One, Two, and Three were printed for the use of the Select Committee on Small Business.
Further citations will be identified by booklet and page

Note 96.
Page 126, Paragraph 2
Senator Bob Dole was in Kansas but he sent a letter . . .
Part 15, Vol 1. p. 5924.

Note 97.
Page 127, Paragraph 2
Dr. Louis Hellman
Part 15, Vol 1. p. 6195.

Note 98.
Page 127, Paragraph 3
that provoked reporter Morton Mintz
"The Pill and the Public's Right to Know" *Progressive* Magazine, May 1970, pp. 25–27

CHAPTER 9: LADIES' NIGHT OUT

Note 99.
Page 130, Paragraph 2
"It's important to explain," Alice reflects today
See Alice J. Wolfson, "Clenched Fist, Open Heart" pp. 268–283 in *The Feminist Memoir Project; Voices from Women's Liberation,* Ed. Rachel Blau Du Plessis and Ann Snitow. New York: Three Rivers Press, 1998.

For more on the 1970 Senate Pill Hearings and Alice Wolfson's role, see the National Women's Health Network web site at www.womenshealthnetwork.org, and film documentaries such as "The American Experience Presents The Pill," a Steward/Gazit Production for *The American Experience*, which first aired on PBS Feb. 24, 2003.

Also see, from Canada, The Canadian Film Board and CBC's production *The Pill* by Erna Buffy, 1999. Both include footage of the demonstrations.

Also see Watkins *On The Pill* (op. cit.,) especially Ch 5, "Oral Contraceptives, and Informed Consent".

Note 100.
Page 131, Paragraph 2

Dr. Marvin Legator, pp. 5042–5960 part 15, Vol. 1.

Dr. David Carr, Professor of Anatomy, McMaster University, Hamilton, Ontario, pp. 600–609 part 15, Vol. 1.

Note 101.
Page 134, Paragraph 3
His first witness, Dr. Hilton Salhanick . . .

Dr. Hilton Salhanick, Professor of Obstetrics and Gynecology, Harvard University, pp. 6381–6391 part 15, Vol. 1.

Note 102.
Page 135, Paragraph 2

Dr. Philip A. Corfman, Director Center for Population Research National Institute of Child Health and Human Development, NIH

Note 103.
Page 136, Paragraph 3
He had married his college sweetheart

Eunice Luccock Corfman grew up in Shanghai where her parents were Presbyterian missionaries. At her death, aged 52 in March 1980, she was chief of the Science Reports Branch of the National Institute of Mental Health. She won an O Henry award for one of her short stories, "To Be An Athlete," about a woman tennis player, and published a novel, *The Roaring Shock Test*, in 1968. The Corfmans are parents of one daughter and three sons.

CHAPTER 10: IF THE TRUTH BE TOLD

Note 104.
Page 137, Paragraph 3
Kistner . . . a witness for the drug industry in pill cases

Kistner's testimony, on Thursday, Jan. 15 appears on pp. 6062–6086. Part 14, Vol. 1.

His unforgettable statement on the difference between a side effect and a complication appears on p. 6082.

CHAPTER 11: ALICE KEEPS BUSY

Note 105.
Page 143, Paragraph 2
Flyers advertising the Women's Hearings on the pill
The Women's Hearings were covered by Alex Ward of the *Washington Post* and other media, and Senator Nelson gave the Wolfson women some space in the Hearing Records. Appendix 10 of Part 17 Vol. 3., reproduces their statements and questionnaires. pp. 7283–7295

Note 106.
Page 144, Paragraph 3
Senator McIntyre's press release including his letter appears in Part 16, Vol. 2., p. 6825

Note 107.
Page 144, Paragraph 5
What could have gone wrong?
The articles from which the quotes from the *New York Times, Washington Post, Washington Star,* and other sources can be found in Part 16, Oral Contraceptives Vol. 2. pp. 6822–6837.

The reporters included here are: Judith Randall from the *Evening Star,* Morton Mintz from the *Washington Post* and *The Progressive,* Victor Cohn from the *Washington Post,* Stuart Auerbach from the *Washington Post,* as well as the *New York Times* and *Science News* unsigned. The announcements of the watering down began on March 24 with AP story in *New York Times* and Auerbach in the *Washington Post.* Victor Cohn on June 24 said that the AMA has promised "a legal and legislative battle against a printed warning due in every package of birth control pills." Sad to say, 33 years later they still will not support it, for reasons discussed in Ch. 6, the "off-label" matter.

Note 108.
Page 146, Paragraph 3
The story behind the sticker
Roy Hertz, M.D., then aged 60, was Associate Director of the Population Council and Senior Physician at Rockefeller University in 1970 when he testified at the Senate Hearings and then—in collaboration with Corfman and Wolfson—came up with a strategy to save the Pill warning. Hertz held many high posts in science research and in academia. He was highly respected for his candor and his principles, and his abiding concerns about estrogen and cancer. He died in 2002, living just long enough to learn about the outcome of the Women's Health Initiative study, which he had predicted.

Note 109.
Page 148, Paragraph 3
See the first FDA protest and the Network's first action at
http://www.womenshealthnetwork.org/ nnartic.les/fdaprotest.htm

Note 110.
Page 150, Paragraph 4
Cindy Pearson . . . charged sexism
She spoke on June 14, 1990 at the Fertility and Maternal Health Drugs Advisory Committee Meeting. She opened her statement with a referral to the Health Network Demo in 1975: "On December 19, 1975 the National Women's Health Network joined by many individual men and women, held a demonstration at the front entrance of the FDA building. We held that demonstration to protest the hazards of estrogen related drugs to protest the FDA's failure to protect the public from the indiscriminate use of hormones. Those demonstrations were motivated by the publication only 11 days earlier, of two *New England Journal of Medicine* articles linking estrogen use to the sharply increased incidence of endometrial cancer. The expression of women's anger on that day in 1975 led to a new FDA requirement that women using estrogen products be given written information.

"Today, almost fifteen years later, we hope that our expression of anger and concern leads to a constructive response from FDA. Premarin has not been adequately studied, and it would be premature to approve this new indication." She was right. I don't know how it happened that she was right and the important doctors on the Advisory Committee were wrong, but it might be something to think about.

Note 111.
Page 150, Paragraph 3
Dr. Bruce Burlington testified that . . . do not constitute randomized prospective clinical trials
The testimony of Dr. Burlington and Dr. Solomon Sobel at the Senate Labor and Human Resources/Aging Subcommittee Hearing was reported on April 29, in the F/D/C report, also know as the "Pink Sheet."

CHAPTER 12: GETTING TO THE HEART OF THE MATTER: ESTROGEN, HEART DISEASE, AND THE TRIUMPH OF SUGGESTION OVER SCIENCE

Note 112.
Page 162, Paragraph 3
"Estrogen and Your Arteries," *Harvard Women's Health Watch*, July 1995, p. 6

Note 113.
Page 164, Paragraph 2
Wellness Facts, The University of California at Berkeley Wellness Letter, Vol. 13, Issue 2, November 1996, p. 1

Note 114.
Page 164, Paragraph 3
"Estrogen-Progestin Combo Benefits the Heart", *University of Texas Lifetime Health Letter*, March 1995, p. 6

Note 115.
Page 164, Paragraph 3
Based on a *Journal of the American Medical Association* Report on the PEPI trial

Note 116.
Page 164, Paragraph 4
"Heart Disease in Women: Special Symptoms, Special Risks," *Consumer Reports on Health*, May 1997, p. 54

Note 117.
Page 165, Paragraph 2
Seaman, Barbara, "The Media and the Menopause Industry," *Extra!*, 1997

Note 118.
Page 166, Paragraph 2
Journal of the American Medical Association, August 19, 1998

Note 119.
Page 166, Paragraph 3
Pettiti, Diana, Accompanying Editorial, *Journal of the American Medical Association*, August 19, 1998

Note 120.
Page 167, Paragraph 1
"Does Estrogen Really Protect the Heart?," *Consumer Reports on Health*, November 1998, p. 11

Note 121.
Page 167, Paragraph 2
"Update on Estrogen and the Heart: Does Hormone Replacement Therapy Protect or Hurt the Heart," *The Women's Health Advisor*, April 1999, p. 3

Note 122.
Page 167, Paragraph 3
"HRT and Your Heart," *The New England Journal of Medicine*: Health News, May 2000

Note 123.
Page 167, Paragraph 4
Dr. Rossouw was one of the head doctors at the Women's Health Initiative

Note 124.
Page 167, Paragraph 4
Colins, Peter, M.D., Nanette K. Wenger, M.D., Jacques E. Rossouw, M.D., and Rodolfo Paoletti, M.D., "Cardiovascular and Pulmonary Disease," *Women's Health and Menopause: A Comprehensive Approach*, International Papers, 2002

CHAPTER 13: HEALTH IN THE BALANCE:
UNDERSTANDING BONES, BONE LOSS, AND NEW METHODS
OF OSTEOPOROSIS PREVENTION AND TREATMENT

Note 125.
Page 169, Paragraph 1
Love, Susan, *Dr. Susan Love's Hormone Book*, Random House, New York, 1997, p. 97

Note 126.
Page 169, Paragraph 2
"Bone Density Testing: Who Needs It, and When?," *Mayo Clinic Women's Health Source*, September 2001

Note 127.
Page 170, Paragraph 1
World Health Organization Guidelines, 1994

Note 128.
Page 170, Paragraph 2
The National Women's Health Network, *The Truth About Hormone Replacement Therapy*, Prima Publishing, Roseville, California, 2002

Note 129.
Page 170, Paragraph 3
Watkins, Elizabeth Siegel, "Dispensing with Aging: Changing Rationales for Long Term Hormone Replacement Therapy, 1960–2000," *Pharmacy in History*, Vol. 43 (2001), No. 1

Note 130.
Page 171, Paragraph 4
Dr. Susan Love's Hormone Book

Note 131.
Page 173, Paragraph 2
"Low Bone Density May Predict Risk of Stroke," *Mayo Clinic Women's Health Source*, August 2001

Note 132.
Page 174, Paragraph 4
Wallis, Lila, general information about Osteoporosis

Note 133.
Page 176, Paragraph 5
Lane, Joseph M., and Lisa Langer, "Preventing Fall: Better Balance Through Tai Chi."

Note 134.
Page 179, Paragraph 1
The Mayo Clinic, 1996

Note 135.
Page 179, Paragraph 2
Bissinger, Marjorie, "Exercise for Bone Health," www.healthology.com

Note 136.
Page 180, Paragraph 2
"Longevity Facts," *The Johns Hopkins Medical Letter: Health After 50*, May 1998, Volume 10, Issue 3

Note 137.
Page 180, Paragraph 2
"Wellness Made Easy," *The UC Berkeley Wellness Letter*, April 1998

Note 138.
Page 181, Paragraph 1
See: www.hnrc.tufts.edu/about/director.shtml

Note 139.
Page 181, Paragraph 2
"Don't Overlook Vitamin D for Osteoporosis Prevention," *Environmental Nutrition*, May 1998

Note 140.
Page 182, Paragraph 5
"More Help, Less Harm with Effective Steroid Use," *The Johns Hopkins Medical Letter: Health After 50*, September 2001

Note 141.
Page 182, Paragraph 2
"Potassium Rich Foods Can Help Offset High Salt Diet Contribution to Osteoporosis," University of California, San Francisco, May 23, 2002

Note 142.
Page 183, Paragraph 1
"Our Readers Ask: Steroids and Osteoporosis," *Johns Hopkins Medical Letter—Health After 50*, April 1997

Note 143.
Page 183, Paragraph 2
"Stand Up to Osteoporosis: Your Guide to Staying Healthy and Independent Through Prevention and Treatment," The National Osteoporosis Foundations, 1995—revised 1999, p. 8

Note 144.
Page 183, Paragraph 2
   The New England Journal of Medicine, October 2001

Note 145.
Page 183, Paragraph 3
   "More Help, Less Harm With Effective Steroid Use," *The Johns Hopkins Medical Letter: Health After 50,* September 2001

Note 146.
Page 184, Paragraph 1
   "Our Readers Ask: Steroids and Osteoporosis," *Johns Hopkins Medical Letter—Health After 50,* April 1997

Note 147.
Page 184, Paragraph 2
   Dr. Susan Love's Hormone Book

Note 148.
Page 184, Paragraph 3
   Journal of Bone and Mineral Research, June 2002, 17:963

Note 149.
Page 185, Paragraph 1
   The National Women's Health Network, *The Truth About Hormone Replacement Therapy,* Prima Publishing, Roseville, CA, 2002

Note 150.
Page 185, Paragraph 4
   "RX News: Treating the Depressed Elderly: Heading for a Fall," Health Facts, October 1998

Note 151.
Page 186, Paragraph 2
   "Osteoporosis: The Hormone Connection," *Health News,* June 2001

Note 152.
Page 186, Paragraph 2
   Annals of Medicine, April 3, 2001

Note 153.
Page 186, Paragraph 3
   "Osteoporosis and High Blood Pressure," *The Women's Health Advisor,* February 2000

Note 154.

Page 186, Paragraph 4

"Laid Up? You're Probably Losing Bone," *Environmental Nutrition*, January 1996

Note 155.

Page 187, Paragraph 1

The National Women's Health Network, *The Truth About Hormone Replacement Therapy*, Prima Publishing, Roseville, CA, 2002

Note 156.

Page 187, Paragraph 3

Seaman, Barbara, "Taking Control of Your Health," *Hands On! 33 More Things Every Girl Should Know*, Suzanne Harper, Ed., Crown Publishers, New York, 2000, p. 148

Note 157.

Page 188, Paragraph 2

Bauer, Douglass C., M.D., "Young Women With Anorexia Nervosa at High Risk of Fracture," Medscape Coverage of the 1st Joint Meeting of the International Bone and Mineral Society and the European Calcified Tissue Society, June 2001, www.medscape.com

Note 158.

Page 188, Paragraph 3

Coney, Sandra, *The Menopause Industry*, Hunter House, Alameda CA, 1994, Pg. 161

CHAPTER 14: LOSING OUR MINDS TO HORMONES:
THE PREMATURE PRESCRIBING OF ESTROGEN FOR
ALZHEIMER'S DISEASE

Note 159.

Page 191, Paragraph 3

Shenk, David, *The Forgetting*. Doubleday, New York, 2001

Note 160.

Page 193, Paragraph 3

Mount Sinai School of Medicine: Focus on Healthy Aging, February 2002

Note 161.

Page 194, Paragraph 2

The Mayo Clinic Health Letter, October 1996

Note 162.
Page 194, Paragraph 3
  Franzen, Jonathan, "My Father's Brain," *The New Yorker*, 2001

Note 163.
Page 196, Paragraph 2
  "Postmenopausal Estrogen and Estrogen-Progestin Use and 2 Year Rate of Cognitive Change in a Cohort of Older Japanese American Women," *The Journal of the American Medical Association*, June 12, 2000, Vol. 160, No. 11

Note 164.
Page 196, Paragraph 3
  Fertility and Sterility, December 2001

Note 165.
Page 197, Paragraph 2
  The Journal of the American Medical Association, March 21, 2001

Note 166.
Page 198, Paragraph 1
  "Effect of Estrogen on Brain Activation Patterns in Postmenopausal Women During Working Memory Tasks," *The Journal of the American Medical Association*, April 7, 1999, Vol. 281, No. 13

Note 167.
Page 198, Paragraph 2
  The American Journal of Epidemiology, October 2001, 154: 733–739

Note 168.
Page 199, Paragraph 2
  Paganini-Hill & Henderson, "Estrogen Deficiency and the Risk of Alzheimer's Disease in Women," *American Journal of Epidemiology*, August 1994

Note 169.
Page 200, Paragraph 1
  The Journal of the American Medical Association, May 1993

Note 170.
Page 200, Paragraph 2
  The Lancet, August 17, 1996: 429–432

Note 171.
Page 200, Paragraph 2
  "Fighting Alzheimer's With HRT," *The Harvard Health Letter*, 1996

Note 172.
Page 200, Paragraph 2
"Alzheimer's and Estrogen: The Latest," *Harvard Women's Health Watch*, November 1996, Vol. IV, No. 3

Note 173.
Page 200, Paragraph 3
Neurology, June 1997, Volume 48, Number 6

Note 174.
Page 201, Paragraph 2
The Women's Health Initiative findings, 2000

Note 175.
Page 201, Paragraph 3
"Reproductive Period and Risk of Dementia in Postmenopausal Women," *Journal of the American Medical Association*, March 21, 2001, Volume 285, No. 11

Note 176.
Page 201, Paragraph 3
The Women's Health Advisor, 2001

Note 177.
Page 201, Paragraph 4
"Postmenopausal Estrogen Replacement Therapy and the Risk of Alzheimer's Disease," *Archives of Neurology*, March 2001, Volume 58

Note 178.
Page 202, Paragraph 1
"Hormone May Help Alzheimer's Symptoms," *The New England Journal of Medicine—Health News*, December 31, 2001

Note 179.
Page 202, Paragraph 2
Journal of the American Medical Association, February 23, 2002, Volume 288, No. 1

Note 180.
Page 203, Paragraph 4
"Current Concepts in Mild Cognitive Impairment," *Archives of Neurology*, December 2001, Volume 58, Number 12

Note 181.
Page 207, Paragraph 4
Morris, John C., "Alzheimer's Disease: Unique, Differentiable, and Treatable," The 52nd Annual Meeting of the American Academy of Neurology, April 29, 2000

Note 182.
Page 204, Paragraph 1
Neurology, May 1, 2001

Note 183.
Page 206, Paragraph 1
"Stroke: A Cause of Dementia You Can Do Something About," Mount Sinai School of Medicine: Focus on Healthy Aging, February 2002

Note 184.
Page 206, Paragraph 1
"Heart Bypass Surgery Associated With Cognitive Decline," *Duke University News,* February 1, 2002

Note 185.
Page 210, Paragraph 3
Journal of the American Medical Association, February 12, 2002

Note 186.
Page 207, Paragraph 1
The Journal of Neuroscience, January 15, 2002

Note 187.
Page 207, Paragraph 2
Environmental Nutrition, February 1997

Note 188.
Page 207, Paragraph 3
"Alzheimer's Cause May Be Metals Buildup," *The Wall Street Journal,* June 21, 2001

Note 189.
Page 207, Paragraph 4
The New England Journal of Medicine, February 14, 2002

Note 190.
Page 208, Paragraph 1
Journal of the American Medical Association, April 26, 1995

Note 191.
Page 208, Paragraph 1
"Gene Linked to Accelerated Brain Again in Healthy Adults," Duke University Medical News, February 25, 2002

Note 192.
Page 208, Paragraph 2
"A New Strategy for Alzheimer's Disease," *The Harvard Health Letter,* January 2002

Note 193.

Page 208, Paragraph 3

"A Vaccine for Alzheimer's?," *The Harvard Health Letter,* January 2002

Note 194.

Page 208, Paragraph 3

"Alzheimer's Treatment Trial is Temporarily Suspended," *The Wall Street Journal,* January 21, 2002

CHAPTER 15: AND BEAR IN MIND . . .
SWIMMING IN THE SEA OF ESTROGENS

Note 195.

Page 210, Quote 1

Landes, Lynne, "A World Awash In Hormones," www.commondreams.org, July 29, 2002

Note 196.

Page 210, Paragraph 1

Long Island Breast Cancer Study Project, Cancer Control, and Population Science, National Cancer Institute, www.epigrants.cancer.gov/libcsp

Note 197.

Page 211, Paragraph 3

Sharpe, R.M., and N.E. Skakkebaek, "Are Oestrogens Involved in Falling Sperm Counts and the Disorders of the Male Reproductive Tract?" *Lancet,* 1993, 341; 1392–95

Note 198.

Page 211, Paragraph 4

Fink, D.J., DES Task Force Summary Report, Washington, D.C., Government Printing Office (DHEW publication No. NIH 79–1688), 1978

Note 199.

Page 212, Paragraph 1

Seaman, Barbara, and Gideon Seaman, M.D., *Women and the Crisis in Sex Hormones,* Bantam, New York, 1977

Note 200.

Page 216, Paragraph 2

Pollan, Michael, "This Steer's Life," *The New York Times Magazine,* March 31, 2002, section 6

Note 201.

Page 216, Paragraph 3

Lean, Geoffrey, and Sadler, Richard, "Male Fertility Fears Over Pollution In Water Supply: Oestrogen In Rivers Makes Fish Change Sex And Poses Potential Risk To Humans," *The Independent,* March 17, 2002

Note 202.
Page 217, Paragraph 2
    Raloff, Janet, "Environmental Concerns Reemerge Over Steroids Given to Livestock," *Science News*, January 5, 2002, Volume 161, No. 1

Note 203.
Page 217, Paragraph 3
    Sower, S.A., K.L. Reed and K.J. Babbitt, "Limb Malformation and Abnormal Sex Hormone Concentrations in Frogs," Environmental Health Perspectives, November 2000; 108(11): 1085–90

Note 204.
Page 217, Paragraph 3
    Nagler, J.J., J. Bouma, G.H. Thorgaard, and D.D. Dauble, "High Incidence of a Male-Specific Genetic Marker in Phenotypic Female Chinook Salmon From the Columbia River," *Environmental Health Perspectives*, January 2001; 109(1): 67–9

Note 205.
Page 218, Paragraph 1
    Pharmaceuticals, Hormones, and Other Organic Wastewater Contaminants in U.S. Streams: Buxton, H.T., and Kolpin, D.W., 2002 U.S. Geological Survey Fact Sheet FS-027-02

Note 206.
Page 218, Paragraph 1
    Schiffer, B., A. Daxenburger, K. Meyer, and H.H. Meyer, "The Fate of Trenbolone Acetate and Melengestrol Acetate After Application As Growth Promoters in Cattle: Environmental Studies," *Environmental Health Perspectives*, November 2001, 109(11): 1145–52

Note 207.
Page 218, Paragraph 2
    Information on Louis J. Guillette, www.zoo.ufl.edu.ljg

Note 208.
Page 218, Paragraph 3
    Hogan, Michael, "Germans Close Tainted Feed Farms," Reuters, July 18, 2002

Note 209.
Page 220, Paragraph 1
    Fagin, Dan, "Tattered Hopes," *Newsday*, July 30, 2002

Note 210.
Page 221, Paragraph 1
    Davis, Devra, *When Smoke Ran Like Water*, Basic Books, New York, 2002

INDEX